T0144681

BASIC HEALTH PUBLICATIONS

USER'S GUIDE

TO NATURAL TREATMENTS FOR LYME DISEASE

Learn How Nutritional and Other Therapies Can Help You Control Your Symptoms.

JAMES J. GORMLEY AND
CAREN FEINGOLD TISHFIELD
JACK CHALLEM Series Editor

Series Editor: Jack Challem
Editor: Roberta W. Waddell
Typesetter: Gary A. Rosenberg
Series Cover Designer: Mike Stromberg

Basic Health Publications User's Guides are published by Basic Health Publications, Inc.

ISBN: 978-1-59120-177-9 (Pbk.)
ISBN: 978-1-68162-865-3 (Hardcover)

CONTENTS

FOREWORD

I would like to personally thank James Gormley and Caren Feingold Tishfield for having written this book to help spread important information regarding one of the most misdiagnosed diseases of our time.

In 1994, my daily activities, which included playing sports outside, lying on the grass in the park, and simply walking across the lawn to get to a nearby swimming pool, were no different from those of millions of other people. Yet, as a perfectly healthy twenty year old, without any rash or other indication that I had been bitten by a tick, I suddenly began having a myriad of strange, unexplainable symptoms. From flulike symptoms, migraines, and partial paralysis, to joint pain, cardiac trouble, and overall malaise, I was becoming sicker and sicker.

Unfortunately, these symptoms mirrored those of many other illnesses, as Lyme disease so often does. After finally getting the correct diagnosis eight months later, I embarked on a very long journey to treat Lyme disease and the other tick-borne diseases that I had contracted.

Due to my own ongoing battle with this illness, in 2002 my husband and I decided to create a foundation called Turn the Corner, which is dedicated to the support of research, education, awareness, and innovative treatments for Lyme disease and other tick-borne diseases. We work hard to educate the public and physicians alike, and to create worldwide awareness of this disease and the integrative healing options that are available, which is why this book is so important.

In this book, James and Caren do an amazing job of defining Lyme disease and its significance as well as providing powerful and actionable prevention methods, and health-boosting treatment choices to help those who have been infected resume their normal lives.

As someone who has had Lyme disease for twelve years, I would encourage all of you to read this book carefully and share the knowledge with your children and the people you love. It is the sort of health empowerment embodied in a book such as this that may just keep this disease from robbing many people of the health and quality of life they treasure.

—Staci Grodin
President, Turn the Corner Foundation
www.turnthecorner.org

PREFACE

The *User's Guide to Natural Treatments for Lyme Disease* is an indispensable resource for people trying to make their way through the briar patch of chronic Lyme disease, which is one of the most challenging and controversial medical disorders encountered in the United States today. First, the guide presents a balanced view of the enormous differences of opinion among physicians on criteria for diagnosis, optimal dosage, and duration of antibiotic therapy. Second, this guide emphasizes the importance of integrating self-care with medical care. A health-promoting, anti-inflammatory diet must be a cornerstone of any healing program. If you are receiving prolonged antibiotic therapy, your diet must also be mindful of the food intolerances and problems of yeast overgrowth that can complicate antibiotic treatment.

Before developing experience with chronic Lyme disease, I had spent years practicing and teaching nutritional medicine and environmental health. Many of the patients I treated were experiencing health problems created by excessive use of antibiotics. Helping people overcome antibiotic side effects and avoid unnecessary antibiotic treatment was (and continues to be) an important part of my medical practice.

Several years ago, I realized that some patients in my care were infected with *Borrelia* or other tick-borne organisms. These patients were often surrounded by disagreements about their diagnoses. Typically, a doctor specializing in Lyme and related diseases (a Lyme-literate physician) had made a diagnosis of Lyme disease, and a rheumatologist or infectious disease specialist at a university-affiliated medical center had disputed it, based primarily upon the results of laboratory tests.

Most of the time, I discovered, the outcome of treatment would eventually indicate that the Lyme-literate doctor was right and the university specialist was wrong. As much as I had been an advocate of caution in the use of antibiotics, I realized that in order to serve my patients well, I had to advocate for the use of antibiotics, often at high dose and for prolonged periods, in appropriate cases.

I turned to established Lyme-literate physicians for advice and found that it was always given generously and thoughtfully—there were very few big egos in this community of doctors. I was gratified to learn that most Lyme-literate physicians had developed a keen interest in nutritional medicine as a support for the treatments they were prescribing. The integration of nutritional and herbal therapies, many of which are described in this *Guide*, with advanced use of conventional medication, has been a great asset to the care of people with late-stage Lyme disease.

My personal experience as a physician has led me to the following conclusions about the role of Lyme disease in chronic illness:

1. Lyme is great at masquerades. If there is a reasonable likelihood that Lyme disease is present, it is usually worthwhile treating, rather than waiting for diagnostic certainty.

2. There is no best treatment regimen for everyone. Individuality rules. The best results are achieved by a flexible and patient-centered approach.

3. People can recover fully from chronic Lyme disease. The horror stories posted in Internet chat

rooms are worst-case scenarios, not typical out-
comes.

4. Lyme disease often leaves a trail of biochemical
and immune system problems in its wake. Curing the infection may not cure the effects of
chronic inflammation. Integrative therapies play
a critical role in helping the resolution of inflammation and restoring normal function to the
metabolism, immune system, and nervous system. Furthermore, for some people, cure of infection can only occur after these areas have
been addressed.

5. The ultimate challenge is knowing when antibiotic treatment can be stopped without a risk of
relapse. Your physician needs your close attention and active participation to make the right
decisions at this stage. Your observations and
opinions are crucial to a successful outcome in
the Lyme disease endgame. Learn to know your
body and understand your symptoms.

The doctor alone cannot cure you.

—Leo Galland, M.D.
Foundation for Integrated Medicine
http://mdheal.org

INTRODUCTION

In 2003, Joan Hansen, a first cousin who lives in Weston, Connecticut, asked me (JG) if I would ever consider writing a book about Lyme disease that included good information about holistic and complementary approaches.

Since Joanie, her husband, Bill, and their children were all affected with Lyme disease to one extent or another, I made a promise to her to gather good, take-home information—along integrative lines—and distill these insights and options into the form of a little book with a big purpose.

In March 2005, another one of us (CF) entered the picture, bringing both clinical nutritionist credentials and personal experience with Lyme disease symptoms that were helped by nutritional supplementation.

Thus our book was born.

During our research into both direct treatments for Lyme disease (such as antibiotic therapy) and complementary support (such as high-potency probiotics), we uncovered many therapies, for both treatment and relief of symptoms. We decided to focus more on those approaches that are believed to be profoundly safe, are in widespread use, and have an established basis in evidence-based practice.

This is not to say, however, that if an alternative therapy is not covered, or is mentioned only briefly, it is not safe. Nevertheless, we chose to err on the side of caution while, at the same time, providing detailed, powerful holistic and integrative support solutions for people with Lyme disease.

Although we titled our book, *User's Guide to Natural Treatments for Lyme Disease,* we consider that any multi-pronged, comprehensive approach to Lyme disease—from using antibiotics to attack the bacterium transmitted by a tick, to improving symptoms and supporting the body's defenses via innovative dietary supplementation and thoughtful use of alternative health modalities—falls under the broad term of *treatment.* We do not mean by this, however, that taking supplements or homeopathic tinctures is going to treat or cure Lyme disease, or that these options, however helpful and powerful, should be used in place of first-line antibiotic therapy.

In fact, we encourage all readers who believe that they, or someone they care for, has Lyme disease to find a licensed, Lyme-literate physician and work with that practitioner in selecting, incorporating, and monitoring the success of the supplements and other integrative choices outlined in this book.

In Chapters 1 and 2 of this *User's Guide to Natural Treatments for Lyme Disease,* we talk about Lyme disease and provide some tips to assist you in determining if you might have the disease, in order to help you prepare before you run (not walk) to a Lyme-savvy physician. Once Lyme disease is diagnosed, Chapter 3 offers a detailed overview of first-line antibiotic therapies—first conventional, then integrative. In Chapter 5, you'll find case reports from people who found success with supportive complementary and alternative approaches, from neurobiofeedback, to acupuncture, to dietary supplementation. One of us (CF) outlines her own personal Lyme disease odyssey in Chapter 6. In Chapter 7, you'll get some good info on avoiding those nasty ticks in the first place (to help prevent initial or repeat infection). Finally, in

Chapter 8 we provide insights on diet and supplementation.

Although no one book can serve as the be-all and end-all of Lyme books, it is our deepest hope that this small book will provide some big benefits in terms of insights, options, help, and support to all people who have been touched by the Lyme disease epidemic.

CHAPTER 1

WHAT IS LYME DISEASE?

What if we were to tell you there is a devastating illness that masquerades as multiple sclerosis (MS), arthritis, and brain cancer, and can cause meningitis, congestive heart failure (CHF), depression, schizophrenia, and a host of other psychiatric disorders? And that 93 percent of those with chronic fatigue syndrome (CFS) and most of those with fibromyalgia have this disease?

What if we were to tell you that Dan Kinderleher, M.D., estimates there are 18 million cases of this disease in the United States alone, and that others estimate there are nearly 1 billion people worldwide who are infected with the organism that causes this disease?

This disease exists, and it is called Lyme disease.

Lyme Disease—Its Discovery

In 1883, the first recorded case of Lyme disease was noted by Alfred Buchwald, who described it as a degenerative skin disorder now known as acrodermatitis chronica atorphicans (ACA). In 1909, Arvid Afzelius presented his research on an expanding ringlike lesion, *Erythema migrans* (EM), linked to what would later become known as Lyme disease. In 1921, Afzelius suggested that the disease might be transmitted by the *Ixodes scapularis* tick, better known as the deer tick.

By the 1940s, people were going to their family doctors with signs of a similar tick-borne illness that usually started with the ringlike rash and then developed into multi-system illness. Later in the same decade, spirochete-type structures were found in skin samples, which led to the use of penicillin as a treatment.

Familiar with these cases, a doctor in Wisconsin diagnosed a patient with the EM rash and successfully treated it with penicillin in 1969. In 1975, Polly Murray and Judy Mensch—two mothers who were alarmed by how many people in Lyme and East Haddam, Connecticut, had crippling, joint inflammation—contacted public health authorities. A group of scientists led by Yale University rheumatologist, Dr. Allen Steere, identified what was then called *Lyme arthritis* in thirty-nine kids and twelve adults.

Many of these people had arthritis, swollen painful joints, headaches, and other neurological symptoms. About 25 percent of them reported having had a bull's-eye (EM) rash with a raised red ring and a clear center around the time the symptoms began to show up. Early treatment with penicillin not only shortened the duration of the rash but also reduced the risk of developing arthritis. Clinical symptoms and environmental conditions suggested this was an infectious disease probably caused by a tick.

In 1982, the spirochete, a type of thin, spiral-shaped bacteria, was identified in the mid-gut of the adult deer tick, *Ixodes dammini* (originally referred to as *Ixodes scapularis*) and was given the name *Borrelia burgdorferi* (Bb) after Willy Burgdorfer, Ph.D., M.D., who discovered that the Bb bacterium was the probable cause of Lyme disease.

It is known today that Lyme disease is caused by one of several hundred known strains of the parasitic bacterium, *Borrelia burgdorferi*, that are transmitted to people by the bite of infected ticks.

In fact, conclusive proof that Bb causes Lyme disease came in 1984 when spirochetes were cultured from the blood of people with the EM rash, from the rash lesion itself, and from the cerebrospinal fluid (CSF) of an individual with meningoencephalitis who had had the EM rash.

The exact type of *Borrelia* infecting people in the United States is called *B. burgdorferi sensu stricto*. Two related *Borrelia*—*B. garinii* and *B. afzelii*—cause Lyme disease in Europe; in fact, in Asia, it is believed that only these two strains cause Lyme disease in humans.

Bacilli
Varying kinds of bacteria classified according to their different shapes, which can be spherical (coccal), rod-like (bacillary) or spiral/helical (spirochetal) in form.

Evidence is building to suggest that some of these parasitic spirochetes specialize in the effects they cause. For example, arthritis appears to develop more frequently following infection with the Bb spirochete. At the same time, neurological problems are more common in infections with *B. garinii*, and skin conditions occur more frequently in connection with *B. afzelli*.

The U.S. Centers for Disease Control and Prevention (CDC) began surveillance for Lyme disease in 1982, and the U.S. Council of State and Territorial Epidemiologists (CSTE) designated Lyme disease as a nationally notifiable disease in 1991.

Why is Lyme disease running rampant today? Environmental change is one reason. According to the National Institutes of Health (NIH), "Urbanization, road and dam construction, deforestation ... and pollution can all play a role in diseases such as Lyme disease."

"One important contributing factor to Lyme disease emergence," says the NIH National Institute of Environmental Health Sciences, "is fragmentation of forest habitat" into tracts smaller than five acres. In addition, species diversity appears to play a role. The more types of animals, including squirrels and opossums, the less incidence of disease there is; the less animal diversity, and the greater numbers of shrews and white-footed mice, for example, the greater the incidence of disease.

A Tick by Any Other Name

In the Northeastern and North Central United States, black-legged ticks (*Ixodes scapularis*) are responsible for transmitting Lyme disease bacteria to humans; on the Pacific Coast, the Western black-legged tick (*Ixodes pacificus*) is to blame.

These carrier ticks, called vectors by disease experts, feed on scores of mammals and birds which, in turn, infect other ticks. During the tick's life cycle, it goes from eggs, to larva, to nymph (it is during these stages that most human Lyme disease transmission occurs), to adult.

Ticks' two-year life cycle favors certain seasons over others for the transmission of new Lyme infections. Its life cycle begins with the eggs being laid in early spring; each female can be expected to lay approximately 3,000 eggs, usually in a pile of leaf litter. The larvae hatch in summer and take their first feeding; this is probably when they first acquire the spirochete infection. Over the fall they molt into nymphs, which take their first meal over the following spring or summer. These nymphs molt into adults over that next fall, feed in the following spring, and then drop off and lay their eggs for the next generation's life cycle to start.

Tiny but Dangerous

Ixodes ticks are much tinier than regular dog and cattle ticks; in their larval and nymphal stages they are no larger than a pinhead. They feed by inserting their mouths into the skin of a host and slowly taking in the blood. It is believed that a tick must be connected to a human host for anywhere from four to thirty-six hours to transmit the Lyme disease bacterium. In addition to its super-tiny size, what also makes these ticks difficult to detect is that they inject a natural painkiller into the skin when they bite (puncture) and when they finally dislodge (withdraw).

The deer tick feeds on humans, small mice, deer, and other animals it is able to latch on to. After latching on, the deer tick takes a blood meal and, in so doing, transmits the Lyme-disease-causing spirochetes to the animal's bloodstream. The tick must remain attached for as long as two to three days in order to take a complete meal, and it is able to transmit the spirochetes during this time.

In addition to deer carriers, experts now also believe that infected ticks are also getting a free ride via about 100 species of migrating birds, not to mention other non-deer carriers, including: chipmunks, foxes, hedgehogs, rabbits, sheep, voles, and the white-footed mouse.

The Risk and Prevalence of Lyme Disease

In the United States, Lyme disease is mainly concentrated in states that are in the Northeastern, mid-Atlantic, and upper North-Central regions, and to several counties in Northwestern California.

Although estimates of the disease's prevalence suggest there are 18 million Americans with the disease and nearly 1 billion people infected worldwide, in 2003 there were only 21,273 cases of Lyme disease reported to the CDC. Although more than 157,000 cases have been logged since 1982, it is known that there is considerable underreporting.

More than 90 percent of the reported cases were from the Northeastern and North-Central United States. The mid-Atlantic region (not New England) did worst, with 14,016 cases, followed by New England (4,079), South Atlantic (1,370), East North-Central (914) and West North-Central (609).

Most of the cases were from the following states, listed by highest-incidence down:

1. Pennsylvania (5,730)

2. New York, upstate (5,179)

3. New Jersey (2,887)

4. Massachusetts (1,532)

5. Connecticut (1,403)

6. Wisconsin (740)

7. Rhode Island (736)

8. Maryland (691)

9. Minnesota (474)

10. New York City (220)

11. Delaware (212)

12. Virginia (195)

13. New Hampshire (190)

14. Maine (175)

15. North Carolina (156)

It was a surprise to both of us when we saw that upstate New York received almost four times the number of reports as Connecticut—that's an eye-opener for a lot of people, especially New Yorkers.

States and territories which had no reported cases were: Arkansas, Colorado, Montana, North Dakota, Oklahoma, American Samoa, Guam, the Northern Mariana Islands, and the Virgin Islands.

Internationally, *Borrelia*-infected ticks and Lyme disease have also been found in Australia, Austria, Bulgaria, Canada, China, the Czech Republic, France, Germany, Great Britain, Japan, Russia, Slovenia, Sweden, and elsewhere.

According to Denise Lang in her book *Coping with Lyme Disease*, "Lyme disease has been called the fastest-growing epidemic of the twentieth century, now surpassing AIDS."

The overall reported-incidence rate of Lyme disease in the United States is 7.39 per 100,000 people, underreporting aside, compared to 3.2 per 100,000 in 1993. According to Lang and other advocates, the CDC acknowledges that the 21,273 cases may represent only 5 to 10 percent of the actual cases of Lyme due to non-reporting by physicians and to the stringent reporting criteria, which apply to under 40 percent of Lyme cases across the board. With these factors in mind, the actual prevalence of Lyme disease could be anywhere from 240,000 to 480,000 cases nationwide.

As far as who is hit by Lyme disease, people of all ages and both sexes are at similar risk, although the highest attack rates are in adults aged forty to sixty-four and in children from age five to fourteen.

In terms of reported cases, the worst Lyme months are July (4,094), August (4,032), December (2,282), September (2,195), and June (2,136). The high incidence in December was a surprise to us.

But we don't want Lyme disease to be a surprise to you. That's why, in the following chapters, we'll help you reduce your exposure to the ticks that carry the disease. We'll also help you find out if you have Lyme disease. If you or someone you care about does, we'll not only share the conventional treatments with you, but we'll also focus on the nutritional, holistic, and complementary approaches that are available.

CHAPTER 2

DO I HAVE
LYME DISEASE?

Whether or not you remember having been bitten by a tick, it is very important to immediately contact a licensed physician if an unusual rash appears on your body.

If you can't get to your doctor's office right away, Karen Vanderhoof-Forschner, cofounder of the Lyme Disease Foundation, recommends the following:

- Mark the outer edge of the discolored rash area with a pen;

- Take a photograph immediately and again two or three days later so you can document the rash's expansion.

An *Erythema migrans* (EM) rash is the only sign that, by itself, allows your doctor to diagnose Lyme disease with certainty. If you don't have the bull's-eye rash, but do have other symptoms of the disease, you need to first ask yourself these questions:

1. Do I have signs and symptoms of Lyme disease?

2. Do my Lyme disease tests suggest I have Lyme disease?

3. Do other tests suggest either another disease or condition, or another illness that has manifested itself at the same time?

4. Have I been exposed to Lyme-disease-transmitting ticks while walking, hiking, or otherwise being in an area known to be tick-infested?

If I Have a Weird Rash . . .

The calling card of Lyme disease is most often a characteristic bull's-eye rash (EM), accompanied by other symptoms, such as fatigue, fever, headache, joint aches (arthralgia), malaise, and muscle aches (myalgia).

The incubation period from infection to the start of the telltale rash is usually seven to fourteen days, but can be as short as three days or as long as thirty days. Some people who have been infected have no recognized illness or have only non-specific symptoms, such as fatigue, fever, headache, and myalgia.

Lyme Disease Progression

Lyme disease typically presents in three distinct stages. Each stage is marked by different signs and symptoms.

Stage 1—Early Localized Infection

Lyme disease spirochetes spread from the tick bite location by cutaneous (skin), lymphatic, and blood-borne routes. The signs of early spread usually show themselves days to weeks after the rash appears. In addition to multiple secondary rashes, diseases related to the heart, the musculoskeletal system, or the nervous system often occur during this period.

Stage 1 disease symptoms typically hit within one to thirty days after being bitten by the deer tick, *Ixodes scapularis* or *Ixodes pacificus*. In this stage, the pathogen, *Borrelia burgdorferi,* begins replicating (making copies of itself) in tissues next to the site of the initial infection.

The signs and symptoms of early infection can include:

- Arthralgia (joint pain);
- Bull's-eye rash (EM);
- Fever;
- Headache;

- Myalgia (muscle pain);
- Neck stiffness (nuchal rigidity).

Erythema migrans (EM) is the most common symptom, occurring in as many as 75 percent of the infected people—it is considered pathognomonic, a defining characteristic for Lyme disease. The rash lesions (or spots) are often circular and reddish, usually not raised, and not always itchy, although they were in my (CF's) case, with the sizes of the rash varying from quite small (1 centimeter) to up to 70 centimeters in diameter. The bull's-eye formation occurs less than half the time; in fact, one of us (CF) had two oval-shaped patches. The rash can show up either at the site of the bite, as seen in 20 percent of those infected, or near it.

The other symptoms (arthalgia, fever, headache, and myalgia) are non-specific for Lyme disease infection and occur in about half those infected. Neck stiffness occurs in something less than half a percent of them.

Stage 2—Early, Disseminated Lyme Disease

Stage 2 Lyme disease occurs within weeks to months of the bite as the *Borrelia* move in the bloodstream from the site of infection to more distant tissues and organs.

Arthritis, cardiovascular, and neurological symptoms emerge at this stage, and symptoms often involve the peripheral nerves, but not those of the central nervous system—the brain, optic, and spinal-cord nerves. Neurological problems are usually marked by Bell's palsy (paralysis of the facial muscles), numbness, pain, visual disturbances, and weakness, or meningitis (brain infection) symptoms, such as a fever, a severe headache, or a stiff neck (nuchal rigidity).

Meningitis

Inflammation of the membranes (meninges) that cover the brain and spinal cord. It is most commonly caused by bacterial, fungal, or parasitic infection.

Other problems, which may not happen for weeks, months, or years after a tick bite, include decreased concentration, irritability, memory and sleep disorders, and nerve damage in the arms and legs.

Signs and symptoms of stage 2 Lyme disease include:

- Cranial neuropathy (abnormal functioning of the cranial nerves in the head);

- Intermittent inflammatory arthritis;

- Meningitis, photophobia (intolerance of or sensitivity to light), phonophobia (fear of, or sensitivity to, sound and speaking), stiff neck.

Meningitis is one of the most common symptoms of stage 2 disease. Neuropathies often affect the seventh cranial nerve and cause facial palsies, especially in children, and may be bilateral (on both sides of the face). Arthritis occurs in about 20 percent of the affected people and usually involves the knee joint.

Musculoskeletal symptoms can include joint and muscle pain that travels from one spot to another; cardiac problems may include myocarditis (infection of the heart muscle) and transient heart blocks (delay in electrical impulses through the atrioventricular node of the heart).

Stage 3—Chronic Lyme Disease

Stage 3, or chronic Lyme disease, can occur from months to years after the tick bite. Infection of the central nervous system causes more severe neurological symptoms. Stage 3 symptoms can disappear for months or years at a time.

Symptoms of stage 3 Lyme disease include:

- Anxiety;

- Ataxia (uncoordinated movements, especially when walking or reaching);

- Atrioventricular conduction abnormalities (AV heart block);

- Brain dysfunction or disease (encephalopathy);

- Decreased memory;

- Depression;

- Mood changes;

- Rheumatoid arthritis;

- Sleep disturbances.

Rheumatoid arthritis (RA) is the most common symptom at this stage and occurs in almost 80 percent of those infected; it typically involves large, weight-bearing joints, such as the knee. Chronic malfunction of many peripheral nerves throughout the body (polyneuropathy) can also develop at this stage, which is usually marked by mental (cognitive) dysfunction, sleep disturbances, fatigue, and personality changes.

Not surprisingly, psychological effects due to encephalopathy and other problems are also very common. Anxiety, depression, and memory loss are typical.

Atrioventricular (AV) block comes and goes at this point, and usually goes away on its own, not requiring pacemaker implantation.

Heart Block and the AV Node

In first-degree heart block, the atrioventricular node (AV node)—which is the tissue between the atria and ventricles of the heart that conducts normal electrical impulses from the atria to the ventricles—has become dysfunctional or diseased and conducts electrical impulses slower than it should. Isolated first-degree heart block is thought to have no clinical consequence, there are no signs or symptoms of it, and there is believed to be no danger of progression to complete heart block.

Current Testing

In the United States, the Food and Drug Administration (FDA) has cleared, or approved, seventy blood tests (serological assays) to help in the diagnosis of Lyme disease. Below is a list of some of the tests used (FDA-recommended or not).

- BAT (Borreliacidal antibody test). In a recent trial of this test's accuracy, the quick BAT assay gave more accurate results than the CDC-sanctioned two-tier system, and for a much lower cost.

- C_6 Lyme peptide test. This test that received FDA approval in 2001 is sensitive and specific enough that other confirmatory tests may not be needed.

- ELISA (Enzyme-linked immunosorbent assay). In this test recommended by the Lyme Disease Foundation, enzymes are used to detect *Borrelia* antibodies. This test is often confirmed with Western blot.

- IFA (Indirect fluorescent antibody). Although prone to error, it is still being used, sometimes to confirm ELISA results.

- PCR (Polymerase chain reaction) test. Although the new generation of this test, called nested PCR tests, appears to be better than the first iteration, this test is prone to a high degree of false-negatives, especially in blood and urine.

- Prevue test. This rapid, in-office test requires only a drop of blood and about thirty minutes to develop. Studies suggest it can detect approximately 50 percent of early Lyme disease; the test is usually confirmed by ELISA or Western blot *and* ELISA.

- Western blot. This procedure—having a positive ELISA result combined with a follow-up Western blot test that is also positive according to very narrow CDC criteria—makes up the current two-tier testing system now in place. The CDC considers Western blot, all by itself, to be 99 percent accurate, although experts still disagree.

In general, Lyme disease is diagnosed in a symptomatic person using a variety of tests. Indirect enzyme-linked immunosorbent assay (ELISA) testing for Lyme specific antibodies in serum is the most common test for Lyme disease. By six to eight weeks after infection, most symptomatic people (96 percent) have detectable levels of anti-Lyme immunoglobulin M (IgM). False positives can be caused by infection from several other diseases, including lupus, rheumatoid arthritis, Rocky Mountain spotted fever, or syphilis.

Blood Serum
The liquid non-blood component of blood plasma in which blood cells are suspended, minus clotting factors; non-blood serum is also found in many other bodily fluids.

Serum immunoglobulin G (IgG) levels require longer (four to six months) to peak than IgM, but are more specific for Lyme. Both IgM and IgG levels remain high long after initial infection even if the disease is not present. IgG titer can remain high indefinitely after exposure.

Early treatment of the disease using antibiotics lowers the serum titer of anti-Lyme antibodies and may contribute to the high (32 percent) false-negative rate that happens with these tests. Western blot (WB) and indirect fluorescent antibody (IFA) assays are used to confirm positive ELISA tests.

Immunoglobulin (Ig)
Any one of the proteins of animal origin having known antibody activity that are found in plasma, spinal fluid, urine, and other body tissues and fluids. Examples are immunoglobulin G (IgG) and immunoglobulin M (IgM).

Cerebrospinal fluid (CSF) cultures obtained by LP (lumbar puncture) are used to confirm Lyme as the cause of meningitis. This test is only positive in 10 percent of those with Lyme disease, however.

The CDC recommends testing initially with a sensitive first test, either the ELISA or the IFA tests, followed by testing with the more specific Western blot test. Although polymerase chain reaction (PCR) testing in serum or CSF has been used successfully as well, this test has not yet been standardized for routine diagnosis of Lyme disease.

The upshot? Consider being tested with ELISA, then obtaining confirmation with, BAT, C_6 testing, or Western blot.

Both the CDC and the FDA say to be careful of labs and tests. In a February 11, 2005 advisory, the CDC and FDA say they have become "aware of commercial laboratories that conduct testing for Lyme disease by using assays whose accuracy and clinical usefulness have not been adequately established."

Antigen (Ag)
Any substance that elicits an immunological response, such as the production of an antibody specific for that substance.

According to the CDC, these not-yet-established tests include urine antigen tests, immunofluorescent staining for cell-wall-deficient forms of *Borrelia*, and lymphocyte transformation tests.

In addition, some labs do polymerase chain reaction (PCR) tests for Bb DNA on the wrong specimens for that test, such as blood and urine, or interpret Western blots using criteria that have not yet been validated and published in peer-reviewed scientific literature.

These inadequately validated tests are also being used to evaluate people in Canada and Europe, according to reports from the Public Health Agency of Canada, the British Columbia Centres for Disease Control (Canada), the German National Reference Center for Borreliae, and the Health Protection Agency Lyme Borreliosis Unit of Great Britain.

In the same advisory, the CDC reminded health-care practitioners that a "diagnosis of Lyme disease should be made after evaluation of a patient's clinical presentation and risk for exposure to infected ticks and, if indicated, after the use of validated laboratory tests."

Get Tested

Moral of the story? If you or your doctor think you've been bitten and you have any of the symptoms, play it safe and get tested (see Testing Resources below); together you can rule out other conditions and causes along the way.

Testing Resources

A number of labs we have run across are:

- IGeneX, Inc. (www.igenex.com) (1-800-832-3200);

- IMUGEN Inc. (www.imugen.com) (1-800-246-8436);

- LabCorp (www.labcorp.com) (1-888-611-3438);

- Specialty Laboratories (www.specialtylabs.com) (1-800-421-7110);

- Inverness Medical Professional Diagnostics (Wampole) (www.invernessmedicalpd.com/clinical/default.asp) (1-800-257-9525);

- Zeus Scientific (www.zeusscientific.com) (1-800-286-2111).

CHAPTER 3

FIRST-LINE TREATMENT— ANTIBIOTIC THERAPY

The best treatment for Lyme disease is, of course, prevention—not getting it at all. But before looking at complementary and integrative approaches to Lyme disease, it's important to get a sense of what the conventional treatment protocol is, if in fact such exists. It really doesn't, and the fact that there is no one single, universally agreed upon—hence definitive—treatment protocol for Lyme disease says something about the chimeral aspect of the disease, something about medications (choice of drug therapy, dosage, and how it's given), and something about people (based on each person's tolerances, sensitivities, and age).

The moving-target nature of the disease is, writes Denise Lang in *Coping with Lyme Disease*, "the crux of the controversy that has polarized doctors, . . . and insurance companies, and sent ailing patients on lengthy searches for relief."

It is known that the *Borrelia burgdorferi* spirochete can hide its appearance, can shape-shift into a cystlike form to evade antibiotics, and can, like syphilis, go into a dormant period, when the person doesn't really feel the symptoms, only to re-emerge later, along with a relapse of symptoms.

While it is true, according to the Lyme Disease Foundation, that "no definitive treatment regimens have been determined, and failures occur with all (approaches)," it is also true that most experts—including conventional, integrative, and holistic practitioners and advocates—recommend, begrudgingly or freely, antibiotic treatment as a first-line therapy.

The National Institutes of Health (NIH) has funded several studies on the treatment of Lyme disease. These studies have shown that most people can be effectively cured with a few weeks of oral antibiotics, especially if the disease is diagnosed quickly and the treatment is started shortly after contracting it.

The NIH National Institute of Allergy and Infectious Diseases notes that early acute Lyme borreliosis is "easily cured by conventional antibiotic therapy" (if treated with the appropriate dose of medication and for adequate time), except for those who develop "various neurological symptoms several months after getting what "appeared to have been successful antibiotic therapy."

Although there are probably many who might be skeptical about the NIH comments on how easily Lyme disease can be cured, the U.S. Centers for Disease Control and Prevention (CDC) agrees with this assessment, remarking that people with neurological or cardiac symptoms related to the disease "may require intravenous treatment with drugs such as ceftriaxone or penicillin." In fact, the CDC says those who are treated with antibiotics in the early stages of infection usually recover quickly and completely, but some, mainly those diagnosed with later stages of the disease, may have symptoms that resist treatment and keep returning. The CDC suggests that these people may benefit from a second four-week course of therapy, although they also note that "longer courses of antibiotics have not been shown to be beneficial and have been linked to serious complications." Fortunately, studies in women who were infected with Lyme disease during pregnancy suggest no negative effects on the fetus "if the mother receives appropriate antibiotic treatment for her Lyme disease," says the CDC.

What Can I Expect with Antibiotics?

People who have tried three-day herbal cleanses and constitutional homeopathic remedies already have a sense of what it feels like to experience a healing crisis, which is a period of feeling worse before you feel better while the body is attempting to eliminate toxins and detoxify itself.

In the same way, before you begin an antibiotic approach (or any approach) to Lyme disease, you should be aware of what people in the Lyme-disease community refer to as a herx or a Herzheimer, also known as die-off syndrome, a detox reaction, or, as mentioned, a healing crisis. Technically known as the Jarisch-Herxheimer reaction, it is a temporary worsening of symptoms that follows widespread killing of bad bugs (pathogenic microorganisms and the toxins they release when destroyed), which, in the case of Lyme disease treatment, lets you know when dead or dying *Borellia* microorganisms (and toxins) are being processed and eliminated by the body.

According to Marc Fett's *Lyme Strategies: Practical Research on Lyme Infection,* Herxheimer effects often include:

- Anxiety, depression, or panic attacks;

- Chills or cold sweats;

- Diarrhea;

- General malaise;

- Headaches;

- Joint or muscle aches;

- Nausea;

- Sore throat;

- Sweating and fever;

- Temporary overall worsening of existing symptoms.

The Herxheimer reaction can be "discouraging

to patients as they progress" on antibiotic therapy and "may be better viewed as a 'good sign' that the bacteria are successfully being killed off," according to Westport Medical Arts, in Connecticut. Dr. Leo Galland, founder of the Foundation for Integrated Medicine in New York, said that, "Resting, drinking enough fluids to avoid dehydration, using treatments that relieve (herx) symptoms, and hanging in there are the best things to do." He adds that it's also important to "definitely let your doctor know what's going on" if you're experiencing what you believe is a herx reaction.

It's fair to say that while there is no be-all and end-all approach to Lyme disease, since each person and his or her disease and response to it (and to treatment) is unique, there are still, nonetheless, generally accepted rules of thumb among mainstream, conventional physicians about how to treat anyone who has been diagnosed with Lyme disease. That said, the first-line treatment is, almost without exception, antibiotic therapy.

Antibiotic Treatment for Lyme Disease

After a tick bite, *Borellia* spreads rapidly, and can be found within the central nervous system as soon as twelve hours after entering the bloodstream. "This is why," according to Lyme-disease-literate, advanced-medicine-pioneer Joseph J. Burrascano, Jr., M.D., "even early infections require full-dose antibiotic therapy" with a medication that is able to "penetrate all tissues" in concentrations known to be deadly to the *Borrelia* organism.

For people who have a visible *Erythema migrans* (EM) rash and begin treatment right away, typical conventional treatment involves up to one month of oral antibiotics, possibly followed by a course of intravenous (IV) antibiotics.

According to "Practice Guidelines for the Treatment of Lyme Disease" from the Infectious Diseases Society of America that were issued in 2000, a standard, conventional course of treatment looks something like the following.

Early Lyme Disease

- For adults: doxycycline 100 milligrams (mg), twice daily (Vibramycin—contraindicated during pregnancy), amoxicillin 500 mg, three times daily for fourteen to twenty-one days, or cefuroxime axetil 500 mg, twice daily (Ceftin).

- For children: Amoxicillin 50 mg per kilogram (mg/kg) of body weight divided into three doses daily (Amoxil), or doxycycline (for kids over eight years of age) at a dosage of 1–2 mg/kg twice daily, maximum: 100 mg per dose (Doryx, Monodox), or cefuroxime axetil at 30 mg/kg divided into two daily doses, maximum: 500 mg per dose.

- For adults with acute (really bad) neurological disease, such as meningitis or radiculopathy: 2,000 mg via IV daily for fourteen to twenty-eight days, or IV penicillin G at 18–24 million units per day, divided into doses given every four hours.

Late Advanced Lyme Disease

(Affecting the central nervous system or the peripheral nervous system)

- For adults: Ceftriaxone, 2,000 mg once a day IV for two to four weeks (Rocephin).

- For children: Ceftriaxone, 75–100 mg/kg daily, in a single IV dose, maximum: 2,000 mg for fourteen to twenty-eight days.

Enlightened Medicine Approaches to Lyme Disease

As suggested earlier, there is a huge controversy between the conventional medical establishment and Lyme-literate physicians on antibiotic treatment for Lyme disease—how long, how much, how often repeated, and so forth. As also noted, enlightened medicine approaches to Lyme disease by Lyme-literate doctors frequently call for much longer, frequently repeated courses of the right antibiotics. These may, especially for those who have chronic, relapsing disease, make them appear to get better but they eventually experience a relapse of symptoms when off the antibiotics.

Another important point is that, as crucial as antibiotic therapy is in treatment for Lyme disease, one huge failing of a *Borrelia*-only approach is a lack of acknowledgement (or understanding) of the fact that people with chronic Lyme disease are almost universally co-infected with other tick-borne nasties at the same time. According to Dr. Burrascano, "These patients have been shown to potentially carry *Babesia* species, *Bartonella*-like organisms, *Ehrlichia, Anaplasma, Mycoplasma*, and viruses."

Studies have shown, explains Dr. Burrascano in the 15th edition of his now-classic monograph, *Advanced Topics in Lyme Disease: Diagnostic Hints and Treatment Guidelines for Lyme and Other Tick-Borne Illnesses*, that co-infection with other organisms at the same time makes people a lot worse and leads to more organ damage.

Dr. Burrascano adds: "Therefore, real, clinical Lyme as we have come to know it, especially the later and more severe presentations, probably represents a mixed infection with many complicating factors."

That doesn't mean that you shouldn't be as aggressive as possible with Lyme; it means that you and your licensed healthcare practitioner should be as far-reaching and comprehensive as possible in your campaign against Lyme disease and any other bugs that have taken advantage of your immune-compromised state and also set up residence.

Antibiotic Therapy

Early Lyme disease (*Borrelia*) is treated for four to six weeks and late (or advanced) disease usually requires a minimum of four to six months of treatment. Treatment of Lyme usually calls for combinations of antibiotics due to the chimeral, and rapidly spreading deep nature of the *Borrelia* organism.

In *Managing Lyme Disease,* Dr. Burrascano provides the following menu of antibiotic choices, to which we have added recommendations from other Lyme disease alternative-treatment experts:

Amoxicillin (Amoxil)

- Adults: Amoxicillin 1,000 mg every eight hours plus 500 mg of probenecid + colchicines, same schedule (Col-Probenecid and Proben-C);
- Children: Doxycycline 50 mg/kg per day divided into three doses every eight hours;

Dr. Raphael B. Stricker at the California Pacific Medical Center recommends the following:

Doxycycline (Vibramycin)

- Adults: 200 mg twice a day with food; doses of up to 600 mg are often needed—*not* for kids or during pregnancy;

Cefuroxime axetil (Ceftin)—useful for EM rashes in people who also are co-infected with skin ailments

- Adults: 1,000 mg every twelve hours and adjust;
- Children: 125–500 mg every twelve hours based on weight;

Tetracycline (Brodspec, Emtet-500, Panmycin)

- Adults only: 500 mg three times a day—*not* for kids or during pregnancy;

Clarithromycin (Biaxin)

- Adults only: 250–500 mg every six hours plus hydroxychloroquine (Plaquenil) 200–400 mg per day (*see* inset), or amantadine (Symmetrel) 100–

200 mg per day—*not* recommended for kids or pregnant women as first-line therapy for early Lyme disease, but for people who cannot take amoxicillin, doxycycline, or cefuroxime axetil, according to practice guidelines from the Infectious Diseases Society of America.

Telithromycin (Ketek)—Expect strong and quite prolonged Herxheimer reactions; ask your doctor to watch your heart-rate-corrected QTc interval prolongation and liver-enzyme numbers;

• Adolescents and adults: 800 mg once daily—*not* for use during pregnancy;

Augmentin XR 1000 from GlaxoSmithKline—A time-release combination antibiotic made up of amoxicillin and the potassium salt of clavulanic acid

• Adults: 1,000 mg every eight hours, up to 2,000 mg every twelve hours.

Misdiagnosis Led to Years of Ineffective Treatment

The Lyme Disease Network of New Jersey (www.lymenet.org) posted a case report on a person whose Lyme disease was misdiagnosed as rheumatoid arthritis and placed on Plaquenil for eight years, with no improvements. After finally receiving the correct diagnosis of Lyme disease, this person was treated with azithromycin (Zithromax) for five months and was cured.

Pulse Therapy

An advanced antibiotic treatment option recommended by Dr. Burrascano is called pulse therapy, which calls for antibiotics (usually administered via the parenteral route) two to four days in a row per week (as opposed to every day) for a period from ten to more than twenty weeks. This allows for

---

AT A GLANCE

**Oral Antibiotics Favored by
Lyme-Literate Doctors**

- Biaxin or Zithromax *plus* Ceftin or cefdinir (Omnicef) or metronidazole (Flagyl)— Dr. Raphael Stricker
- Doxycycline—Dr. Stricker
- Minocycline—Dr. Stricker
- Rifampin (Rifadin, Rimactane)—Dr. Dietrich Klinghardt
- Zithromax *plus* minocycline combination— Dr. Klinghardt

---

dosage increases of cefotaxime (Claforan), up to 12,000 mg a day. This may be an option when conventional daily approaches have failed.

Combination Therapy

This involves using two or more very different antibiotics at the same time to create synergistic effects and reach different tissues. According to Dr. Burrascano, a typical combination calls for a cell-wall medication plus a protein inhibitor, such as amoxicillin or clarithromycin. The downside of this sort of treatment is stomach upset and bad yeast infections.

How Do I Know if the Antibiotics Worked?

Although medical books suggest that a person is cured of Lyme disease after x number of days of treatment, most healthcare practitioners who treat Lyme disease believe that a person is not cured of Lyme unless two months of symptom-free time has passed.

Antibiotic Therapy—In Perspective

As Dr. Ron Schmid, cofounder of the Alternative Medicine Center of Connecticut, wrote, "When the disease is diagnosed early, when it initially appears, antibiotics are not unreasonable, and often eradicate the organism that is involved in Lyme." He added that, "Many people go this route and never have a further problem." He clarified his perspective on antibiotics, however, by pointing out that once the disease has been established for several months, as was Dr. Schmid's own case, conventional treatment typically calls for months of intravenous antibiotics, where results are, Dr. Schmid notes, "at best mixed."

According to Dr. Dietrich Klinghardt in Bellevue, Washington, "Antibiotics have disappointed in the treatment of Lyme disease" as a stand-alone treatment. "Antibiotics alone will not help us to cope with the coming plagues."

Klinghardt feels, and we believe rightly so, that we all need to "start looking *beyond antibiotics* for help and for hope."

CHAPTER 4

COMPLEMENTARY SUPPORT FOR LYME DISEASE:
DIETARY SUPPLEMENTS

Lyme disease affects the whole body, so why shouldn't the approaches to it show an appreciation of that? According to Steven J. Bock, M.D., "An integrative approach to medical treatment of Lyme disease starts by considering" the entire picture. Dr. Bock, for example, looks at:

- Genetic/hereditary tendencies;

- History of antibiotic treatment and how long each treatment lasted;

- Knowledge of any co-infections;

- Mental state and mood;

- Metabolism;

- Nutritional status;

- Previous immune-function problems or infections;

- Recent disease history and symptoms.

Lyme-literate doctors are also concerned whether the proper antibiotic was used and if it was used long enough. For example, although the conventional medical community usually recommends a four-week course of antibiotics, Bock typically places anyone with an early diagnosis of Lyme disease on a six-week course of antibiotics supplemented with probiotics.

Nutritional Supplements

Probiotics are one example of the key role that dietary supplements play in helping improve the health of people with Lyme disease, from reducing symptoms, to counteracting unwanted effects of medication, to helping rid the body of toxins as detoxification strategies are employed.

What follows are specific nutritional treatment protocols from some of the leading experts who treat people with Lyme disease today. Some of the nutrients are recommended by several different doctors, and we're aware of the overlap, but are presenting the supplements this way for two reasons:

1. You can decide which protocol you want to try (along with your Lyme-literate healthcare professional);

2. We wanted to faithfully present the protocols as we got them. Another good thing about repeating the listing of these nutrients is that you have multiple assurances these supplements are broadly recommended.

According to Joseph J. Burrascano, Jr., M.D., studies of people with Lyme disease have shown that some of the symptoms are "related to cellular damage and deficiencies in certain essential nutrients."

Dr. Burrascano's basic supplementation plan for those with Lyme disease looks something like this:

- B-complex—This is very important for neurological symptoms; Dr. Burrascano says to take one B-complex supplement per day, and if the neuropathy is severe, add 50 milligrams (mg) of vitamin B_6 daily; but he cautions not to take these if you are taking the prescription drug atovaquone (Mepron, Malarone);

- CoQ_{10}—This is important for the heart and also for resistance to infection, 200–300 mg per day;

- Essential fatty acids—These help with aches, concentration, dizziness, fatigue, mood, and weakness; a combination of high-quality omega-3 and omega-6 oils is recommended;

- Magnesium—This is very helpful for "tremors, twitches, cramps, and muscle soreness," says Burrascano; take at least one tablet/capsule daily;

- Multi-vitamin/mineral (high-potency, USP certified);

- Probiotics—These are critical for anyone on antibiotics; shoot for a high-potency probiotic supplement, such as acidophilus, with at least 2 billion colony-forming units (CFUs) per capsule.

In his Alternative Medicine Center of Connecticut, in Watertown, Ron Schmid, N.D., agrees about the importance of essentials fats, and, in fact, specifically recommends high-potency cod liver oil.

Dr. Bock supports the use of fish oil, but also believes that high-quality plant oils are important too. He recommends borage seed oil, to which he adds a high-potency multi-vitamin/mineral and, to address muscle pain and spasms, a calcium/magnesium supplement. Additional magnesium is given if symptoms are fibromyalgialike. He also gives CoQ_{10} and L-carnitine to promote energy, as well as intravenous administration of the B vitamins and vitamin C, partly for "immune function enhancement."

Another antimicrobial (anti-infective) approach is cat's claw (uña de gato), which is recommended by Ron Kennedy, M.D., of Santa Rosa, California. He suggests that people seek out high-quality extracts that are standardized to a minimum of 0.5% pentacyclic oxindole alkaloids (POAs) and are *free* of tetracyclic oxindole alkaloids (TOAs).

To tackle the spirochete infection and any co-infections, Dr. Dietrich Klinghardt, in Bellevue, Washington, uses pulsed electromagnetic field therapy (KMT microcurrent technology); B-complex vitamins, such as B_6 and niacin; herbal extracts, such as forskolin from the Ayurvedic herb, *Coleus forskohlii;* and minerals, such as copper, iron, manganese, magnesium, and zinc.

According to Klinghardt, restoring, or filling up, the body's mineral reserves "has always been the most essential part of our heavy metal detox program . . . It is also the most essential part of our Lyme treatment." On the one hand, Klinghardt focuses on what a person with Lyme symptoms is missing, such as magnesium, and on the other hand, what that person has too much of, such as mercury, compared to someone without the disease.

To address the negative effects of neurotoxins released by Lyme and co-infection organisms, Klinghardt recommends alpha-lipoic acid, apple pectin, beta-sitosterol, chlorella growth factor (CGF), chlorella, essential fats, propolis powder, and raw vegetables.

Dr. Burrascano also targets specific symptoms, and has a list of optional supplements that are indicated for special circumstances.

Neurological Symptoms

- Acetyl-L-carnitine taken along with SAM-e can help with short-term memory; take 1,500 mg of acetyl-L-carnitine on an empty stomach, along with 400 mg of SAM-e daily; although benefits may be seen in as little as three weeks, plan to use the combination for three months or more.

- Methylcobalamin (methyl B_{12}). This prescription drug made from vitamin B_{12} helps heart and muscle function; ask your healthcare practitioner to give you a 25 mg intramuscular injection once daily.

More Antioxidants

- Green tea. Drink several cups of decaffeinated tea daily, or use in extract form.

- *Cordyceps* is known to improve energy and lung function, and to reduce fatigue; it can be used long-term. Look for a brand that provides 1,000 mg of *Cordyceps mycelia* per daily supplement serving.

Immunity

- Echinacea may help with acute and chronic viral infections; three weeks per month for a limited time.

- Reishi may help natural killer cell activity; look for brands that provide 500 mg or more of the active ingredient per capsule.

Joint Support

- *Boswellia serrata*, containing over 400 mg of boswellic acid per daily serving.

- Glucosamine can benefit joint health; fine to use a high-quality product long-term.

Optional Supplements

- Creatine may help with neuromuscular concerns; work with your healthcare professional on a *loading dose* of 20 grams per day for the first few days, then follow label directions afterwards, or work with your healthcare professional on higher doses; make sure to drink plenty of fluids while on creatine.

- Milk thistle helps liver function; shoot for over 500 mg per day.

Leo Galland, M.D., works very hard to individualize each supplementation regimen based on the specific needs of each person with Lyme disease. Dr. Galland agrees with recommendations of other Lyme-savvy doctors and includes injections of two nutrients, magnesium and vitamin B_{12}. Galland's recommendations are especially unique regarding inhaled glutathione, 50 mg, four times per day. Dr. Galland has also had some excellent response to the use of IV glutathione, 1,000–2,000 mg as a *rapid push* twice a week.

Fred Pescatore, M.D., medical director of Partners in Integrative Medicine, New York, agrees with Dr. Galland about glutathione, and additionally recommends active hexose correlated compound (AHCC) for immune-boosting, 500 mg three times a day, indefinitely; N-acetyl-cysteine (NAC) for liver-cleansing, best in conjunction with glutathione, for up to one year per course of treatment; monolaurin, 300 mg per day, for up to one year; oregano, 500 mg three times per day, for up to one year; and intravenous vitamin C, 35–50 grams per treatment for up to three months.

Other Approaches

Many protocols and approaches came across our desks while researching this book—some intriguing, some inspiring, and some downright unusual. Our goal has been to focus on nutritional therapies as an adjunct to an enlightened antibiotic regimen, while making mention of other treatments that are out there, without leading people down dangerous and slippery treatment slopes.

Vitamin C and Salt

One approach that seems to be very popular in some circles—we have each spoken with at least one person who swears by this—is the oral salt and vitamin C protocol, which is 1,000 mg of pure salt (not table salt), 1,000 mg of vitamin C, and glasses of pure water taken at intervals throughout the day. Since the National Research Council has set 2,400 mg of sodium as an upper safe daily limit to avoid kidney or hypertension problems, *this protocol must be fully looked into, researched, and discussed with your Lyme-literate healthcare professional before considering it.*

Homeopathy

Ronald D. Whitmont, M.D., in Rhinebeck, New York, told us that the goal of classical homeopathy is "to treat the patient who is sick, to strengthen the immune system, and to eradicate the illness by supporting the host." Dr. Whitmont has written, "The starting point for homeopathic medical treatment of Lyme disease and other related . . . infections is the history and physical exam." He has noted, "It is important to remember that the diagnosis of Lyme disease does not automatically imply the treatment, homeopathically." However, he says, looking at the homeopathic repertory, the following remedies stand out.

- Arsenicum album
- Carcinosin
- Lac caninum
- Ledum palustre
- Mercurius corrosivus
- Syphilinum
- Thuja occidentalis

In early Lyme, and for prevention, Whitmont recommends the use of classical homeopathy as a first-line treatment. He observed that "The

---

Supplement Must-Haves

Most Lyme-literate experts recommend these supplements:

- Acetyl-L-carnitine
- Antioxidants, including CoQ_{10} and vitamin C
- B-complex, including B_6 and B_{12}
- Chromium picolinate (recommended by CF)
- Glutathione
- Magnesium
- Multi-vitamin/mineral
- Probiotics

judicious use of homeopathic medicines applied through the classical homeopathic approach is one of the best means to cure Lyme disease . . . and to reestablish a healthy equilibrium."

Take Away?

While certain approaches to Lyme disease—including acupuncture, Chinese herbal medicine, neurobiofeedback, and nutritional supplements—have been observed to definitely help people improve their symptoms, Dr. Klinghardt notes that other "treatment modalities have been surprisingly ineffective," including hyperbaric oxygen, ICHT (intercellular hyperthermia), and ozone.

Fortunately, dietary supplements (herbal extracts, minerals, vitamins, and specialized supplements) can be safely and effectively used to support the process of healing, offset unwanted side effects of antibiotic treatment, and tackle the ongoing, sometimes lingering, symptoms and effects of chronic Lyme disease.

Although nutritional therapy is critical to long-lasting, fundamental healing, it is often a slow build, meaning that its benefits are obvious over the long-term, but not right away; in fact, sometimes outward symptoms do not improve until a few months after supplementation is initiated. Provided that acute symptoms are immediately brought to the attention of your healthcare professional, in nutrition-based therapy patience is often rewarded by an improvement in chronic symptoms, and sometimes quite dramatically, as with Peter whose health transformation is chronicled in the next chapter.

CHAPTER 5

COMPLEMENTARY TREATMENTS FOR LYME DISEASE:
CASE HISTORIES

What Antibiotics Destroyed, Natural Therapies Restored

Dr. Rima E. Laibow, medical director of the Natural Solutions Foundation in Croton-on-Hudson, New York, gave this first-person report on how she was able to reverse a steep decline in a formerly vital, active man who had contracted Lyme disease some time back.

Peter called my office and asked if I treated Lyme disease. He had had more than a year of continuous intravenous (IV) antibiotics, but was losing ground with every day that passed.

He had been a successful advertising executive running his own firm when he started to feel fatigued and unwell. Competitive and over-committed, he shrugged off the malaise and aches, which made it more difficult to work or play hard. In his recreational life, Peter had to give up tennis, and was constricted to one activity: sleep.

At work, it became harder to remember details and focus on the requirements of accounts. With no time or energy for anything but the struggle to complete each day's work, his personal life collapsed. He lost his friends and his wife left him. Lack of focus, reduced concentration, and issues with memory sapped his much-valued edge, which dulled to the point that his employees seized his company and forced him out.

With no family, friends, income, or energy, Peter became despondent, though he still searched for a doctor who could get him back to the life he recognized but could no longer live. One new doctor had a nasty shock for Peter: the Lyme spirochete had damaged his heart. But cardiac drugs did not help, and Peter's fatigue increased as his heart struggled to provide enough oxygen to his brain and muscles. The downward spiral continued when Peter lost his sight—his neurological Lyme disease had cost him not only most of his memory and focus, but his vision as well.

That's when Peter called me to ask if there might be some clinical stone unturned. I asked how he would get to my office, about an hour from his home by car, and when he said he would *drive*, I knew he was highly motivated to get well. I also knew his judgment was seriously impaired and helped him make arrangements to get to my office safely.

His medical records were thick, comprehensive, and tragic. Western medicine suppresses symptoms by poisoning enzymes, not by dealing with underlying causes of disease. So, while Peter had been desperately seeking out help, the underlying disease processes that were destroying his organs were never addressed.

When Peter arrived in my office, he was gaunt, feverish, and angry—in pain, yet still determined to get his life back. He was also demanding, mean, and domineering, attempting to bully and control the staff, and totally unconcerned about anyone but himself. Knowing from his history and his records that he had received vast, prolonged courses of IV antibiotic treatment, and believing, as I do, that antibiotics are often highly detrimental to the immune system, I suggested a different course of treatment. I asked Peter if he were willing to change virtually everything because, for a person as ill as he was, there was little time for gradualism. Peter agreed, and we began working together along several different paths at the same time.

Peter's GI tract and bacterial balance had been seriously harmed by so much antibiotic therapy. Approximately 80 percent of the immune system resides in the gut and Peter's was not doing well. His digestion and gut status were dreadful and, since the beneficial bacteria had been wiped out of his gut by the drugs, I asked him to take daily high doses of probiotics (beneficial bacteria), digestive enzymes, and the nutrients necessary for healthy GI and immune function. I also developed a detoxification program he could carry out at home, using such herbs as milk thistle for liver support, along with commercially available detoxification products to remove the toxic burdens on his body from his careless, pre-disease lifestyle, and the huge number of toxic drugs he had taken.

Nutrients support the immune and healing processes of our bodies. Yet, as is sadly typical, none of Peter's previous physicians had considered the nutritional status of his body in their attempts to help it get well. I considered this a major error and began treating Peter with high-density nutrient IVs several times a week. These IVs contained mega-doses of B-complex, vitamin C and other vitamins, selenium, trace and nutritional minerals (including iodine, manganese, magnesium, and zinc), glutathione, and other natural items depleted by his illness and by the treatment he had received over the years of his illness. He, like all biological beings, required additional nutrients for healing and I provided them via the IV route.

At the same time, Peter began a neurological training process called neurobiofeedback (www.nbcb.org). Since Western medicine understands that the brain regulates both function and repair for the entire body, and the technology of neurobiofeedback allows the brain to learn new and better ways of doing just that, I felt certain that this powerful, non-invasive, and self-regulated treatment would offer Peter positive input in his quest to regain his health.

We began with sessions in the office where Peter and his helper were trained in the technique of placing sensors at precisely selected locations on his scalp and earlobes. Once they could do that reliably, Peter began to learn how to control his brainwave (EEG) output through auditory feedback. The computer program listened to his EEG output and rewarded him with carefully tailored sounds when his brain waves assumed the characteristics I was reinforcing during thirty-minute clinical sessions three to five times a week.

When Peter and his aide could perform these tasks perfectly, we provided him with a Nintendo-sized device that he could plug into his computer at home to continue the treatment, without having to make a two-hour round trip every day. We also arranged for his nutrient-dense IVs to be administered at home so he did not have to come to the office more than once a week.

Peter totally changed his diet to eliminate all pesticides, dangerous industrial chemicals, and toxins. His diet became totally organic and was modified to his particular individual needs and sensitivities.

Within a few weeks, Peter's energy level increased dramatically. He was no longer continually fatigued, and was able to carry out a full day's activities without paying the price in bone-deep exhaustion. His mood began to lift rapidly, in part because of his newfound hope (depression is often a consequence of insufficient nutrient density, including a lack of essential fatty acids). Peter's aches, arthritis, fevers, and malaise left him. I continued the IVs and other treatments since I knew that, although Peter was improving steadily and his body and brain were healing, he was by no means out of the woods. I knew that lurking spirochetes were waiting for a favorable moment to come out of hiding again and cause a relapse. I also knew that the negative immune stimulation, which leads to chronic Lyme disease, takes a long time to resolve, and that, despite Peter's newfound robust state, a premature interruption of treatment would be a serious error.

Over time, his ability to concentrate, remember, and plan came back and stayed with him. Peter was beginning to rebuild his business and was reentering his life. He was jubilant. Then one day, he walked into our office—by himself. His vision had come back. There were still times when he was again blind, but his sighted periods gradually grew longer and longer, until there were no dark times, unless his eyes were closed.

The cardiac status took longer to improve but, after about six months, that also began to normalize. Peter continued his treatment with me for about a year, during which time, every system and function that was monitored continued to improve. By the end of that year, all his laboratory tests had normalized, his vision was excellent, his heart was close to normal, and his concentration and mental faculties were sharp and focused. Treatment had been intense and long-term, with nutritional IVs, neurobiofeedback, diet, and supplements, and it had all succeeded, enabling Peter to determine that he was really well—and really busy—so he was ready to terminate therapy.

One more healing had taken place as well. When Peter first came to me, he was determined to get well by dominating his disease, just as he had dominated everyone and everything in his life, but by the time we said goodbye to each other, he was a new man. He had learned to feel sincere appreciation and was able to cooperate, rather than dominate. He had gone from demanding service to working with people, and, most important of all, Peter had learned to love himself and, consequently, love others, too. Peter had become not only well, but *whole*.

Chronic Lyme Disease Subdued with Intense Nutritional/Supplemental Therapy

Helene Richter, the principal of Training through Creative Arts in New York (www.creativetrainingarts. com), discusses the path of her on-again, off-again Lyme disease, and reports on what was done to manage it.

I was originally bitten in 1989. I didn't have any bull's-eye rash and, in fact, I was not diagnosed for two years. From 1991 to 1994, I was treated off and on with oral and IV antibiotics, and from 1994 until 2000, I was fine.

After childbirth in 2000, I started having symptoms, and by September of that year, the symptoms—severe migraines, intense neuropathy, lethargy, and neck pain—had gotten much worse. Once again, I was diagnosed with Lyme disease, this time with two co-infections, for which I was treated with antibiotics.

The treatment was not effective, and by 2002 I had stopped working and was bedridden on IV Zithromax for three months. It worked and I was fine until 2003 when I again relapsed. This time, I was put on the IV antibiotic for four months, and when the symptoms continued, I was put on oral antibiotics.

A minor relapse in 2004 is what led me to Dr. Leo Galland. Instead of antibiotics, he treated me for yeast overgrowth and leaky gut with the natural products Perm A vite from Allergy Research and VSL#3 probiotic from VSL Pharmaceuticals. He also instituted an overall health plan, and recommended a variety of supplements, including:

- Complete Omegas (3,6,9) from Nordic Naturals;

- Metabolic Co-Factor from Allergy Research, and calcium;

- MigreLief from Quantum with feverfew;

- NT Factor from Nutritional Therapeutics;
- Saventaro Cat's Claw from Enzymatic Therapy;
- Super D_3 Vitamin D from Allergy Research.

Around this time, I also began with Caren Feingold at Foodtrainers (www.foodtrainers.net), and was put on a yeast-free diet. The Foodtrainers' elimination diet helped me achieve a dramatic overall improvement in pain levels and lose thirty-five pounds. In addition, bodywork and weekly Pilates classes really helped reduce the pain in my joints and improved my flexibility, strength, and endurance.

With Dr. Joseph Burrascano, I continued on antibiotics, beginning with 800 milligrams (mg) of Ketek daily, but when this caused diarrhea, I reduced the amount to 400 mg a day, five days on, two days off. I also took 500 mg of the natural supplement bromelain, to increase the antibiotic's benefits, and the probiotic Florastoracidophilus, which cleared up my stomach problems.

Dr. Galland had me take the natural supplement glutathione, which improved my pain symptoms immediately by reducing the neuropathy and neck pain. I had two IV pushes done in two months and then began glutathione nasal spray (it smells like rotten eggs, but it worked well).

I feel the best I have since my relapse in 2000. I have maintained my weight loss and am exercising regularly at a local gym. I now have the energy to expand my consulting practice and take on major projects, including teaching, where I stand more than eight hours in front of a roomful of people. I continue to take 400 mg of Ketek, but have reduced my dose to three weeks a month and am continuing to wean myself off this antibiotic.

I am still on a modified food plan that includes very low yeast, and I have eliminated dairy and wheat altogether.

My supplements (and one medication) for maintenance now include, besides those originally recommended by Dr. Galland:

- Candex from Pure Essence Labs, to fight candida;

- Magnesium glycinate, 400 mg, two to four times a day for muscle spasms;

- 1 baby aspirin;

- Probiotics from Custom Probiotics;

- Vitamin C, 1,000 mg in the morning.

Doctor Says Traditional Chinese Medicine (TCM) Cured Her Lyme Disease

Dr. Kathleen Hall, President/CEO (www.DrKathleen Hall.com), was treated by Dr. Clark Casteel with traditional Chinese medicine, including acupuncture and Chinese herbs, and discusses her treatment in this report.

I am a doctor married to a physician, and my daughter is also a physician at Georgetown University Hospital, but that did little to help me when I was first diagnosed with Lyme disease.

I took the standard course of treatment, the antibiotic doxycycline, for sixty days, but continued to have enormous problems. The pain in my legs was excruciating. I couldn't sleep, and would actually cry much of the night. I had memory loss and problems with confusion, and Western medicine could not address any of these long-term complications.

I finally went to Dr. Clark Casteel, a practitioner of traditional Chinese medicine (TCM), and using acupuncture along with his own formula of Chinese herbs, he literally *cured* me of my Lyme disease. Dr. Casteel told me that Western medicine uses a threshold to decide if you are cured from Lyme disease, but that doctors of Chinese medicine know the disease lingers below this threshold within the cells, and that only by accessing the disease at this subcellular level can it really be eradicated.

Dr. Casteel's Comments on TCM

Lyme disease, by nature, creates a pattern in Eastern medicine we would refer to as a blood heat pathogen. Since the pathogenic, or disease-causing, factor goes into the bloodstream, it sneaks around the other defenses the body can use if something bad is digested, for example.

One model for the pathogenic invasion into the body by pernicious or *evil* influences is called the *4 portions model*. This can basically be viewed as varying layers of the body, from outer to inner penetration, by pathogens related to wind heat. It would be erroneous to compare this model directly with modern biomedical concepts of the immune system as it also involves disharmonies in the function of chi (life energy) in immunity, a concept absent from Western medicine. It is interesting to note that one of the main patterns, or symptoms, of a blood-level pathogenic penetration is skin eruptions. This is seen in Lyme disease and in late stages of AIDS, another blood level presentation. When treating for Lyme disease, my strategy consists of acupuncture combined with herbal therapy.

Primarily, the underlying TCM diagnosis is of the utmost importance. This varies according to the varied imbalances inherent in each person. The focus is on restoring homeostasis, and may be influenced in each patient by other health conditions, medications, and emotional issues. The theory in traditional Chinese medicine of *treating the whole person, not the disease,* is strongly supported in my practice.

Typically, however, for those who do not have an active Lyme disease pattern, special attention is given to strengthening chi and building blood, while simultaneously clearing toxic heat from the blood. By eliminating an environment which is suitable for the spread of Lyme disease, the host (the person's body) becomes increasingly inhospitable to its presence.

My Lyme disease herb formula is as follows:

- Ban lan gen (Indigowoad root);

- Bai zhu (Bighead atractylodes rhizome);

- Danggui (Chinese angelica root);

- Gancao (Licorice root);

- Liaoqiao (Weeping forsythia);

- Pu gong ying (Mongolian dandelion herb);

- Tu fu ling (Glabrous greenbrier root).

CHAPTER 6

"I AM IN CHARGE OF MY LYME DISEASE"

What follows is a report on my own (CF) experience with Lyme disease, starting with my coming down with Lyme disease in June 1996 (even though I didn't know I had it then) and progressing to where I am today.

In June 1996, I was visiting a friend in Bridgehampton, Long Island. As friends were busily getting ready to meet their families for a Fathers' Day brunch, I sat outside by the pool, which was enclosed by woods, to soak up the last of the weekend rays.

The next week I developed a flat red rash on my abdomen, which basically followed the bikini line of my bathing suit. There were two oval-shaped patches running diagonally from my hip to my pubic area, which began to itch, prompting me to call my dermatologist. I also woke up that week feeling greatly fatigued and as though I had a hangover. My energy was low and I was anxious and irritable. Aside from the rash, I thought the symptoms were related to my partying weekend in the Hamptons combined with exercising in the heat and being in grad school.

My first stop was a general practitioner (GP). His diagnosis? Sand mites. He asked if I had washed my towels, showered after the beach, and taken other sanitary precautions, all of which I told him I had done. He prescribed lindane (gamma benzene hexachloride, with such brand names as Kwell or Thionex), which I used with no results.

My second stop was the dermatologist's office. I showed her the rash, told her what the GP had diagnosed and prescribed. She said sand mites, too, and gave me a cream and some soap. Again, no change.

By now, other physical and psychological symptoms were mounting. These included constipation, confusion, depression, headaches, an inability to tolerate the heat and sun of summer, a lack of desire or ability to get out of bed in the morning, melancholy, stiffness in muscles and joints, stiff neck, sugar cravings, and a terrible reaction to alcohol.

I knew, rationally and intellectually, something was not right, but I could not pinpoint *what,* since my symptoms were all over the place. Here I was, an active, vivacious, social, athletic, intelligent twenty-six-year-old graduate student in nutrition who, in a matter of three to four weeks, suddenly had a different personality, increased anxiety and depression, an inability to exercise, a lack of desire to socialize, and a change of appetite and taste for foods. I went from eating an extremely healthy diet to desiring only sugar-packed foods.

What was happening? I honestly did not know where to turn. I said to myself, "I think I have Lyme disease," and went to the Internet to research it.

Back at the GP's office, I said I hadn't been feeling well. I described only the physical symptoms. I was too embarrassed to tell him all the other neurological/psychological symptoms I had, as I thought he would consider me crazy. And I, too, thought, maybe if I felt better physically, the emotional stuff would subside.

I told him I suspected Lyme disease, and he asked if I had been in the woods, or had been hiking. I explained I had spent time in Central Park over the summer and had visited friends in the Hamptons. His response was, "There is no Lyme in New York City and, unless you were actually playing in tall grass or in the woods, you wouldn't have gotten it in the Hamptons," concluding, "You have a summer flu and are probably run down."

My next stop was a gastroenterologists's office. By now it was September, and I was more and more confused and less and less able to articulate my thoughts and words. When I went to this GI doctor, he tried to take an in-depth history, but I couldn't keep things in chronological order and ended up sounding demented.

His consensus was, " I'll test you for Lyme even though you most likely do not have it. There's no EM rash, no swollen red joints. In the meantime, I think you should start Prozac—you're single, twenty-six, living alone in New York, and I understand it can be tough on you. I think the constipation is secondary to tension and depression, and this will relax you and the muscles of your GI tract, and ultimately help the problem."

I begged him to not only do an ELISA, but also a Western blot, as I had read about the trouble with these tests not being foolproof. Approximately ten days later, this specialist left a message, "The Lyme tests are negative, as I anticipated. Hope you are doing better with the help of the meds." Later, after being correctly diagnosed, I found out that my test was *not* negative, but borderline, and I should have been re-tested immediately.

By now, my sleep was completely messed up, and all the Prozac did was make me more lethargic. Either I could not fall asleep, or I would awaken in the wee hours of the morning. Prior to this, I had been a great sleeper, actually loved my sleep, and nothing was better to me than a good eight to ten hours' rest at night. I never had insomnia before, never had trouble staying asleep, and would only wake up in the morning when my alarm clock sounded. What was *happening* to me?

My family said it was because I was obsessed that something was the matter with me and was looking for an external answer instead of looking within. I was very angry at them because I had always been totally in tune with my body and absolutely knew something was seriously wrong. When family and friends denied this, I became irate, but did not know where to turn to validate what I instinctively knew.

In the autumn of 1996, I started experiencing heart palpitations, night sweats, and anxiety that made me bounce off the walls. I was also unable to sit still. Impatient and moody, I felt like I was a chicken running around without a head, day in and day out.

In December 1996, my back went out. Of course, everyone said, "You're pushing yourself too hard at the gym." Although I was doing less than ever, I was pushing myself through workouts because at least while I was doing them, they cleared my mind and made me feel better. The MRIs and x-rays I had were all negative, but I had muscle spasms up and down the entire back, buttocks, and legs. Even though I had sciatica-like pain and weakness in my legs, everyone said I was fine. Even my skin was a wreck though. It looked like I was going through puberty again, with breakouts on both my face and back. A new dermatologist prescribed minocycline.

Then I was hit with my first Herxheimer reaction. I had no idea what was happening, and thought I was just really sick for a few days with a bad flu that suddenly subsided. Now I *really* couldn't sleep. I actually think I slept a total of twenty hours in ten days. Then one morning, I got out of the shower and had black and blue marks all over my buttocks and hamstrings. The doctor said, "You must have fallen in your sleep and not realized it." Yeah, right. But now that there was physical evidence, even my family started to show concern.

Enter a Lyme-literate doctor from New York's Lenox Hill Hospital. I *finally* received a diagnosis.

He said an equivocal test, plus all of the symptoms, confirmed that, "You most certainly have Lyme." I re-tested positive. Hallelujah—a diagnosis almost nine months later. I was never so happy to hear I was sick—not that I was happy to have Lyme, but happy to finally know something real was causing my symptoms. If I had something real, I knew it could be attacked medically.

This doctor started me on amoxicillin, and pro- benecid to boost the effects of the antibiotic. He told me to stop reading and researching on the Internet because there was a lot of misinformation out there, and I would be fine after a few months of this treatment. I had a bad feeling, though. Shouldn't I be on IV treatment? After all, I had been sick for over nine months and had several neurological symptoms. I asked about the chances of getting a candida/yeast infection from all the antibiotics. Again, he poo-pooed me, saying that IV therapy was hokey medicine, whereas he prac- ticed *real* scientific medicine, and he asked me again to please stop reading, to just take the med- ication and I would be fine.

My second Herxheimer reaction came with a vengeance. About a week into his treatment, I was feeling sicker than ever—bedridden, sweat- ing, and up all night, with nerve pain shooting throughout my entire body. The tingling nerve pain made me feel as though I had bugs in my body and my bones. The Lenox Hill Hospital doc told me to try and go for a walk as it could ease symptoms. *Walk?* I could barely make it to the bathroom and back to bed. After a few days where I couldn't even get out of bed, the herx symptoms subsided.

Although I was thankful that this doctor had cor- rectly diagnosed my Lyme, I didn't have full faith that he was really treating me as a whole person. His *only* concern was ridding me of spirochetes, and he mostly ignored my attempts to discuss building my immune system by using less invasive, nutritionally oriented adjuncts to treatment.

What to do next? My research led me to Dr. Lesley Ann Fein, a physician in West Caldwell, New Jersey. Finally, a doctor who seemed to get the whole picture. I was having sugar cravings, and rather than tell me it was psychological, she explained why, and suggested a dietary regimen of low sugar, low carbohydrates, and moderately high protein. I started on this diet, and when I followed it religiously, I felt much more balanced. There were fewer wild swings in my blood sugar, my cravings decreased, my sleep improved, and I had renewed energy. *AMAZING!*

Dr. Fein also introduced me to vitamin injections—magnesium for muscle spasms and B_{12} for energy. I think the magnesium was a big help. I also took her specially formulated multi-vitamin/ mineral/herbal formula. It helped a little, but I supplemented it with things I discovered on my own. I cut out all sugar, yeast, simple carbohydrates, and fermented foods, and followed a fairly bland, bare-bones diet, consisting of oatmeal and protein powder in the morning; cottage cheese on rye crackers as a snack; sliced turkey on rye crackers, or yeast-free spelt bread with lettuce, tomato, and avocado at lunch; soybeans for a snack; and broiled fish or chicken, steamed vegetables, and beans or sweet potatoes at dinner. I limited salt, avoided artificial colors and preservatives, and had no alcohol, caffeine, or sugar, and no artificial sweeteners. I lost ten pounds (not intentional or necessary), and looked almost too thin, but felt much better—all this while walking around with an IV in my arm giving me a constant infusion of IV cefotaxime sodium (Claforan).

My next stop was Dr. Leo Galland, the founder of the Foundation for Integrated Medicine in New York and the author of *Power Healing*. I was starting to worry about the effects of long-term antibiotic use and wanted to make sure I was doing *everything* possible to optimize my immune system. Dr. Galland helped me fine-tune my diet to ensure that it was completely yeast-free, sugar-free, and mold-free, and he started me on nystatin—a good, broad-spectrum antifungal antibiotic recommended by anti-candida pioneer Dr. William Crook—stronger probiotics, and an anti-fungal medicine, fluconazole (Diflucan). He also upped my intake of fish oils and magnesium.

Fast-forward four years to 2000. Prior to this time, I had experienced a few periods of wellness only to have them followed by horrific relapses when I got lax on the diet and supplements, and went off antibiotics for a few months. Was this going to be the rest of my life? Couldn't I just get rid of this once and for all?

After a relapse in 2000, I decided to consult with Dr. Joseph Burrascano, the guru of all gurus in the Lyme arena. Dr. B. put me back on IV therapy and added a variety of basic and optional dietary supplements to fine-tune my supplement regimen (*see* Chapter 4). As before, I followed this regimen religiously at first, but popping over twenty-five pills a day can take some getting used to.

Now I come to the present. I continue to wax and wane. I'm better after about a month of high-dose antibiotics, but symptoms start to re-appear when I'm about one to three months off the meds.

I do believe, however, that my diet and lifestyle have played the biggest role in my recovery. When my life gets crazed, harried, and busy (like that of a normal New Yorker), I get run down and become symptomatic. If I loosen up on my eating and dabble in some alcohol and desserts, I start paying the price after a while in increased flulike symptoms, decreased energy, increased fatigue, decreased concentration, a need for more sleep, stomach bloating, constipation, and other debilitating conditions.

If I get stressed out or increase my workload one month, the next month is bound to be a lower-energy month for me. My husband can testify—if I don't get adequate sleep, don't exercise sufficiently, or eat a well-balanced, clean diet—I fall apart. I suppose that, similar to an infant just out of the womb, my system is much more sensitive and fragile than that of the average person without Lyme.

So, over the last several years I have come to terms with the fact that I have to live life *that* much more cautiously, be *that* much more aware, and always think ahead about the health consequences of my actions and behaviors. I continue to be open to new approaches to my Lyme, whether it will be more focus on the yeast overgrowth, or added attention to my blood-sugar control. I try new approaches each month, and each year and will never, ever give up because I have the power over my Lyme. I keep it guessing and off-balance by trying new approaches. I make life difficult for it by sticking to my pro-living and anti-Lyme lifestyle.

So, although I may not ever be able to say with 100 percent certainty that I am *cured,* I can say right now that *I have beaten it.* And I will always will be able to say that, whatever relapses I may or may not have, because *I am in charge*—and always will be.

CHAPTER 7

REDUCING EXPOSURE TO LYME DISEASE

If you live or vacation in the Northeastern, the North Central (especially Wisconsin and Minnesota), or the Pacific coast (especially California) regions of the United States, you are more likely than others to be bitten by a Lyme-carrying tick. In descending order, the top five states with the highest numbers of reported cases of Lyme disease are: Pennsylvania, New York (upstate), New Jersey, Massachusetts, and Connecticut.

Pennsylvania, the leading state for Lyme-carrying ticks, has traditionally had hot spots of ticks in Burks, Chester, Delaware, and Montgomery counties. What is less well known, according to Dr. Richard Dryden at Washington and Jefferson College in Washington, Pennsylvania, is that there are other red-hot spots, including Presque Isle State Park in Erie County (162 of 263 deer ticks collected in 2000 and 2001 were positive for Lyme), and Colonel Denning State Park in central Pennsylvania.

Repeat Bites and Tick Avoidance

According to the University of Maryland Medical Center, prompt treatment with antibiotics is very effective in curing Lyme disease in nearly all infected people, including children. It should be noted, though, that even if Lyme disease has been successfully treated, it may be possible to become reinfected with the disease again at a later date. This risk appears to occur only in people who had been treated for the rash, however. In those who developed symptoms of arthritis as well, the antibody response appears to persist and prevent reinfection.

To help avoid initial or repeat bites from Lyme-infected ticks, the following measures can prove useful, and should be considered:

1. **Avoid tick habitats.** Try to stay away from areas known to be tick havens, especially in spring and summer when nymphal ticks feed. Spots favored by ticks are moist, deer-and-rodent-heavy areas, particularly shaded areas with a lot of leaves on the ground, and low-lying vegetation in wooded, brushy, or overgrown grassy habitats. If you are in a tick-infested area, walk in the center of the trails.

2. **Wear the right clothing.** Light-colored clothing makes it easier to spot ticks and carefully remove them before they become attached. Wearing long-sleeved shirts and tucking pants into socks or boot tops (not fashionable, but important) may keep those nasties away from your skin. Wearing high rubber boots may also provide additional protection, especially since ticks are usually located close to the ground.

3. **Use insect repellents** (*see* list on page 60).

4. **Shower:** Dr. Michael P. Zimring, director of the Center for Wilderness and Travel Medicine at Baltimore, Maryland's Mercy Hospital, said, "Usually it is best to take a shower when getting in from the woods, which would also be a good time for a tick check.

5. **Perform a tick check and remove attached ticks.** Since the transmission of Lyme bacteria is likely to occur within thirty-six hours of a tick bite, daily checks for ticks and promptly removing any attached tick you find will help prevent infection. Ticks should be removed using a fine-tipped tweezer, not with petroleum jelly, a hot match, nail polish, or other products. With the

tweezer tip, grab the tick firmly and as closely to the skin as possible. With a steady motion, pull the tick's body away from the skin. Do not squeeze, crush, or puncture the body of the tick. Although the tick's mouthparts may stay in the skin, don't worry. The Lyme bacteria resides in the tick's midgut or salivary glands. After removal, clean the bitten area with an antiseptic and wash your hands with soap and water. Save the tick (in a small plastic bag) for identification in case you develop symptoms.

6. **Use antibiotics after a tick bite?** According to the CDC, "the relative cost-effectiveness of post-exposure treatment of ticks bites to avoid Lyme disease" in Lyme-prone areas is a personal choice, with your Lyme-savvy doctor, although it is not recommended by CDC. According to Dr. Zimring, however, "I believe there is now documentation that if one gets a 200 mg dose of doxycycline, one can avoid the disease."

7. **Make your property Lyme-unfriendly** (see pages 62–63).

Repelling Ticks

In contrast to true insecticides, insect repellents are not designed to kill, but to either deter the insect from its flight path or cause the insect, such as a tick, to fall off.

The concept of attacking Lyme disease via *prevention* has been gaining a great deal of momentum. According to the Centers for Disease Control and Prevention (CDC), the "principal approach to prevention of vector-borne diseases is avoidance." In fact, an entire organization—Stop Ticks On People, or STOP (www.stopticks.org)—has been established and is "dedicated to the prevention of Lyme disease and other tick-borne disorders by stopping the disease at its source, the tick."

The STOP initiative was created at the recommendation of the Dutchess County Legislative Task Force to Study Tick Control, and carries out its work in partnership with Families First New York (www.familiesfirstny.org). STOP has a mandate to seek, help develop, and promote the use of "safe environmental solutions to tick control," with the goal of "reducing the incidence and prevalence of tick-borne disease through education, research, and prevention."

In line with stopping the disease at its source, many different chemical compounds, systems, and products have been developed to keep ticks at bay. As mentioned, the main approaches to fending off and controlling ticks include:

- Applying repellent lotions or sprays to exposed areas of the skin;

- Applying an insecticide or repellent to clothing, shoes, bed nets, and camping gear;

- Applying a repellent to the perimeter of an area or property line;

- Using bait stations that coat feeding animals (chipmunks, deer, and mice) with an insecticide so the transmission cycle is blocked.

Applying Repellents to Skin

The U.S. Environmental Protection Agency (EPA) has registered several active ingredients for use in personal repellents applied to the skin. These ingredients are found in the following products:

- DEET (N,N-diethylmetatoluamide): Backwoods Cutter, Ben's 30 Tick and Insect Repellent, Cutter Tick Defense, Deep Woods OFF!, Deep Woods OFF! for Sportsmen, Repel Insect Repellent Family Formula, Repel Sportsmen Formula, Sawyer Controlled-Release Insect Repellent, Sun and Bug Stuff Lotion.

- Picaridin (KBR 3023): Cutter Advanced.

- MGK-326 (used with DEET): Cutter Tick Defense.

- MGK-264 (included in MGK-326 formulations): Cutter Tick Defense.

- IR3535: Avon Skin-So-Soft Bug Guard Plus IR3535 (spray or lotion).

- Oil of citronella: All Terrain Herbal Armor, Burt's Bees Herbal Insect Repellent, Buzz Away, Green Ban for People, Natrapel Plus.

- Oil of lemon eucalyptus (p-menthane 3,8-diol): Off! Botanicals Insect Repellent, Repel Lemon Eucalyptus Insect Repellent.

So which are best? Well, there's a lot of debate on that. A good bet is to go with a product that has a moderate level of the active ingredient, says it does not irritate the skin, and has a safety profile with which you feel comfortable.

Applying Insecticides and Repellents to Clothing and Gear

Products containing permethrin come up prominently in this category. Permethrin works as a contact insecticide, damaging the nervous system of insects that come in contact with it, leading either to knockdown or their death. Ticks crawling across permethrin-treated pant legs or socks are likely to drop off before they are able to attach and feed.

Permethrin should be applied to clothing, tent walls, mosquito nets, and so forth, but *not* on the skin, unless you are being treated for scabies or crabs. When treating a garment with permethrin spray, spray the cloth outdoors and allow it to dry before wearing. When applied to clothing, permethrin offers protection lasting up to two weeks or two washings, whichever comes first. Clothing soaked in permethrin solution is effective on stored garments for up to four months per application.

Other Repellents and Ways to Control Ticks

Besides using repellents on yourself, your clothes, and your gear, there are repellents designed to be sprayed or otherwise serve as a tick barrier, and there are bait stations designed to help protect animals from ticks.

Tick Barriers and Bait Stations

Perimeter repellents: Ben's Backyard Formula, Mosquito Barrier, a liquid garlic repellent, or Repel Outdoor Fogger "Camp Fogger."

Small (and large) animal bait stations: The Maxforce Tick Management System consists of a series of bait boxes to lure mice and chipmunks that carry infected ticks on their backs. Passing through, these animals are coated with small amounts of a low-dose insecticide (fipronil) that will kill any ticks the animal is carrying, and will protect it from new ticks for up to forty days. This system is believed to reduce backyard tick populations by 80 percent after one year, and 96 percent after two years.

Deer bait stations: The USDA Agricultural Research Service (ARS) patented what is called the 4-Poster Deer Treatment Bait Station, a system developed at the ARS Laboratory in Kerrville, Texas. The bait station controls ticks feeding on white-tailed deer once the deer rubs one or more of the four tickicide-treated applicator rollers located by the feeding stations; the tickicide is slowly transferred by the treated rollers to the heads, necks, and ears of deer as they feed on the deer food. In tests conducted throughout the eastern half of the United States, the device has been shown to work very well against ticks feeding on deer.

Making Your World Tick Free

In addition to all the tick avoidance-and-control measures we've discussed, you should also consider modifying your home's outside landscape to create tick-free zones that make your property Lyme-*unfriendly*. Ticks need moist environments and die quickly where it's dry, so knowing this you can use a few tricks, such as establishing a drying barrier to cut down on the number of ticks in grassy areas.

Other Tips

- Mow the lawn, clear brush and leaf litter; keep the ground under bird feeders clean, and stack woodpiles neatly in dry areas.

- Keep playground equipment away from yard edges and trees.

- Remove plants that attract tick-infested deer, and construct physical barriers to discourage them from coming near your home.

CHAPTER 8

EATING WITH LYME DISEASE

The previous chapters have focused on treatment, holistic approaches, and supplements to improve health and ease the symptoms associated with chronic Lyme disease. It's now time to look at lifestyle and dietary changes that are helpful in managing the disease and its symptoms.

You already know that what you eat can affect your body's immune and inflammatory status and, in the process, either minimize or exacerbate some of the everyday symptoms of this disease. First and foremost, Lyme disease is considered a disease involving inflammation, which can be beneficial (as when you bump your elbow or cut yourself and the area being healed gets swollen), or harmful (as when you have an infection, or when the body is overcompensating for something it sees as a threat).

It's really important to keep in mind that everyone is different and that, because of individual differences in both the disease and each person's biochemistry, dietary approaches that work for one person with Lyme may not work for another. There is no one-size-fits-all diet, no matter what, so it is important to understand that you have unique nutritional needs and that you need to carefully monitor how you are doing with your diet. This is true whether or not you have Lyme, although getting your diet right is even more critical if you have the disease. In reading through this chapter, keep in mind what you might already know about yourself regarding foods that you feel *work* for you, and foods to which you may be sensitive or allergic.

The Basics

Most Lyme-savvy doctors agree that all those with Lyme disease should avoid alcohol and simple sugars, and limit caffeine. People with Lyme disease tend to feel badly after drinking alcoholic beverages, even in moderation. In addition, sugar and its many friends actually feed the Lyme spirochete. Sugar is also a pro-inflammatory food; it encourages yeast overgrowth and is a burden on the immune system, so it is strongly advised to avoid it or keep its intake to a minimum.

Many people with Lyme experience hypoglycemia or hypoglycemic-like reactions, so a low-sugar hypoglycemic diet is recommended. This also involves eating every three to four hours to help control blood-sugar fluctuations.

Caffeine, another pro-inflammatory chemical, has been known to worsen some of the common symptoms of Lyme, such as anxiety, erratic sleep and sleep disturbances, or even heart palpitations.

In addition to limiting alcohol, caffeine, and sugar, it is important for people with Lyme disease to watch how much they eat every day. People who are actively infected, chronically ill, or experiencing a flare-up in symptoms tend to be less active to begin with, which can put on pounds. And being above your ideal body weight has been noted to make inflammation worse, and exacerbate many of the symptoms associated with Lyme disease.

An anti-inflammatory diet is recommended for anyone with Lyme disease. Inflammation in the body is primarily regulated by a group of hormonelike fatty compounds known as prostaglandins. Some prostaglandins,

Prostaglandins
Physiologically active, fatty hormonelike compounds involved in inflammatory response that are found in a range of different tissues.

such as those from omega-6 seed oils, intensify the inflammatory response while others, such as those from omega-3 oils, reduce it, so you can affect this balance by the type of foods you eat. For example, a diet rich in omega-3 fats from fish oil displaces the omega-6 fats, which are disproportionately overeaten in the standard American diet (SAD).

The easiest way of reducing the production of pro-inflammatory compounds is by avoiding processed foods (boxed, canned, frozen, in a wrapper) and instead eating whole, unprocessed foods in their natural form.

Things to Limit or Avoid in an Anti-Inflammatory Diet

Here are the key steps to follow in anti-inflammatory diet:

1. Limit excess consumption of omega-6 fats and avoid polyunsaturated vegetable oils, such as corn oil, cottonseed oil, or soybean oil.

2. Limit dietary intake of saturated fat—avoid fatty meats, including deli meats and hot dogs, butter, cream, and deep-fried foods.

3. Avoid trans fats and limit foods that contain the partially hydrogenated vegetable oils found in margarine and most processed foods.

4. Avoid sugar. This means all simple sugars, including barley malt, beet sugar, cane juice, cane sugar, high fructose corn syrup, honey, or maple syrup, found in cakes, cookies, pastries, candies, fruit juices, and sodas.

5. Avoid white grains and starches. Limit your intake of low-fiber carbohydrates, such as white bread, white rice, or white potatoes, as well as starchy vegetables, such as corn and peas.

6. Limit packaged and processed foods. They may be convenient, but these items are more often than not loaded with omega-6 fats, sodium,

additives, or preservatives, and people with Lyme disease can be especially sensitive to them.

Things to Include in an Anti-Inflammatory Diet

1. Dietary sources of omega-3 fats: Ample amounts can be found in fish, walnuts, flaxseed oil, hempseed oil, and pumpkin seed oil.

2. Nuts and seeds: Choose raw almonds, raw walnuts, pumpkin seeds, and soy nuts.

3. Vegetables: They are high in antioxidants, so aim to get a variety of color each day by choosing at least one from each group below.

   • Greens—asparagus, broccoli, collards, kale, mesclun, spinach, string beans, zucchini.

   • Orange/red—carrots, orange peppers, red peppers, tomatoes.

   • White—cabbage, leeks, onions, radishes.

4. Fruits: Also high in antioxidants; include one to two servings of low sugar/high-fiber fruits daily. Choose from apples, blackberries, blueberries, grapefruits, kiwis, pears, raspberries, and strawberries.

5. Whole grains: These include high-fiber grains and starches, such as barley, beans, brown or black rice, quinoa, sweet potatoes, and whole-grain crackers. Choose varieties with 3 grams or more of fiber per serving.

6. Choose low-fat sources of protein: Beef (filet mignon or sirloin), fish (coldwater varieties such as Pacific halibut, sardines, or Pacific wild salmon, are safer), game meats (bison, buffalo, ostrich), omega-3 enriched eggs, pork tenderloin, tofu, and white meat poultry.

7. Use seasonings, herbs, and spices: Flavor foods with anti-inflammatory seasonings and spices,

such as cayenne, cinnamon, garlic, ginger, rosemary, and turmeric.

8. Beverages: Stay hydrated. Enjoy (primarily) water, seltzer, tea, especially green tea, and vegetable juices.

9. Choose anti-inflammatory supplements, such as cat's claw, curcumin, ginger, rosemary, St. John's wort, and silymarin (milk thistle extract).

Real-Life Lyme Diet

Eat approximately every three to four hours to avoid getting weak, shaky, or too hungry, as hypoglycemia is prevalent in people with Lyme. If this sounds complicated, it's not. To prove it, here is a sample day to give everyone a one-day snapshot of a real-life diet that anyone can follow.

Caren's Lyme Diet—Sample Day
Breakfast

2 omega-3 enriched eggs, such as Organic Valley or Country Hen organic, a serving of low-sugar fruit (blackberries, grapefruit, kiwi, pears, raspberries), and an optional slice of seven-grain/flax-enriched/yeast-free bread or crackers, such as Pacific Bakery.

Green tea with unsweetened soy milk or organic low-fat milk.

OR

Plain Stonyfield Farm yogurt with berries, coarsely chopped walnuts and/or ground flaxseeds.

Green tea with unsweetened soy milk or organic low-fat milk.

OR

Dr. Leo Galland's Omega Blast Granola (recipe courtesy of Dr. Leo Galland's *The Fat-Resistance Diet*).

1 cup non-fat milk or unsweetened soymilk

3 cups rolled oats

1 cup oat bran

$1/2$ cup coarsely chopped walnuts

$1/4$ cup freshly ground flaxseeds

$3/4$ cup pomegranate juice

2 teaspoons walnut oil or olive oil

1 teaspoon cinnamon

1 teaspoon vanilla extract

1 cup raisins

Preheat oven to 325°F. In a big bowl, mix everything except the raisins. Spread mixture over nonstick baking pan and bake for twenty minutes, or until brown, stirring occasionally to cook evenly. Remove from oven and add in raisins. Let cool and put in a glass container; store in the refrigerator. Makes about 5 cups.

Mid-Morning Snack

Flax crackers—Amy Lyn's is an excellent brand.

OR

Raw almonds or walnuts—While very healthy, calories in nuts do add up quickly, so keep to a small handful, or just under twenty nuts.

OR

Low-fat cottage cheese and high-fiber crackers (Kavli Golden Rye or Scandinavian Bran Crispbread).

Lunch

Leafy salad greens with a can of light tuna or salmon, or chicken or turkey breast—add vegetables of choice, and sprinkle with an olive/flax oil blend and fresh lemon.

Optional—two rye crackers or one slice of seven-grain/flax-enriched/yeast free bread.

OR

Tofu and vegetable stir fry—use sesame oil and fresh garlic.

Optional—brown rice or barley (keep to 1 cup).

Mid-Afternoon Snack

Smoothie—1 scoop unsweetened whey, rice, or soy protein powder, fresh berries, 1 tablespoon ground flaxseeds, soy or skim milk, water, and crushed ice.

OR

1–2 tablespoons all-natural almond butter on celery sticks, pear, or rye/brown rice crackers.

OR

1 cup edamame in pod.

OR

Low-fat cheese and sliced tomatoes.

Dinner

Start with mixed green salad, and a walnut oil and lemon dressing.

OR

1 bowl Immune Power Soup (recipe courtesy of Dr. Leo Galland's *The Fat-Resistance Diet*):

2 cups sliced carrots

1 cup chopped leeks (white and light green parts only)

1 cup chopped celery

1 cup diced onions

4 garlic cloves, minced

1 tablespoon extra virgin olive oil

1 tablespoon peeled, minced fresh ginger

1 cup finely sliced shiitake mushrooms

1 cup chopped fresh parsley

$1/4$ cup chopped fresh basil

1 teaspoon finely grated sea salt

Freshly ground black pepper to taste

$1/4$ cup chopped fresh chives, for garnish

Heat oil in a large pot. Add the carrots, leeks, celery, onions, garlic, and ginger, and sauté for ten minutes over medium heat, stirring frequently.

Add the shiitake mushrooms, parsley, basil, and 8 cups pure water. Season with salt and pepper. Turn the heat to high and bring to a boil; then reduce the heat to medium-low and simmer, covered, for twenty minutes. Serve in a bowl or mug and garnish with chives. Makes 5 servings.

Grilled, broiled, baked, or steamed fish (flounder, sole, tuna, wild salmon) seasoned to taste, with greens (collards, kale, spinach, or a mix) sautéed in olive oil with fresh garlic and ginger, and quinoa.

OR

Baked chicken (preferably organic white meat without skin) seasoned to taste, with broccoli and cauliflower steamed or sautéed in garlic and olive oil, and medium-sized baked sweet potato.

Dessert

Fresh fruit.

OR

Sugar-free, organic dark chocolate.

OR

Handful of nuts.

OR

Cube of low-fat cheese.

OR

Sugar-free/no-sugar-added cookies (good brands: Aunt Gussies, Joseph's).

What If the Anti-Inflammatory Diet Doesn't Seem to Help?

If you are adhering to the above guidelines for an anti-inflammatory diet, but it doesn't seem to be helping, or if you are on high-dose or long-term antibiotics, then it's possible you have a candida overgrowth.

Candida is a yeastlike bacteria that's in everyone's intestinal tract. Normally kept in balance by the immune system and good bacteria, candida can get out of control when you take antibiotics or when your immunity is weakened by bacteria, the environment, viruses, and so forth.

Once candida overgrowth occurs, it starts to take up residence in other tissues of the body. According to people who have a systemic yeast infection (or candidiasis), the symptoms are similar to, and may exacerbate, symptoms associated with Lyme disease, including anxiety, depression, and mood swings; fatigue and lethargy; food intolerances or sensitivities; impaired cognitive function; joint pain; muscle pain; memory loss; and weakness.

In addition, most people with a systemic yeast infection also experience gastrointestinal upset, such as belching, bloating, constipation, diarrhea, or gas, as well as vaginal yeast infections.

Considering a Yeast-Free Diet

If this matches what you're experiencing, then we suggest you adopt a yeast-free, anti-candida diet. While the guidelines may seem too restrictive at a first glance, one of us (CF) has seen the symptoms of Lyme disease improve markedly in those who stick to the plan.

In contrast to the anti-inflammatory diet, in most instances a yeast-free diet is not meant to be lifelong, but rather to serve as a temporary intervention to rid the body of the yeast overgrowth and replenish the good bacteria in the gut.

Depending on how bad your candidiasis is, you may notice an immediate improvement, or it may take up to a month to truly feel a difference. Likewise, some people can follow the guidelines prudently for four weeks and go back to eating according to the anti-inflammatory protocol. Others, especially those who have been on and off several antibiotics over the course of many years, may need to strictly follow the more restrictive yeast-free diet for up to six months and still continue to watch their intake of problematic foods thereafter.

Things to Limit or Avoid in a Yeast-Free Diet

(Adapted from Dr. William Crook's *The Yeast Connection*)

1. Avoid alcohol.

2. Avoid sugar. It doesn't matter if it's honey, maple syrup, dextrose, fructose, glucose, lactose, maltose, sucrose, or any -ose, fruit concentrate, or even fresh fruit—it's all the same to yeast.

3. Avoid vinegar (found in salad dressings, catsup, mustard, pickles, and so forth).

4. Avoid cheese and bread (including pita), most crackers and pretzels, yeast extract (found in many commercial soups, bouillons, and sauces).

5. Avoid dried fruits, commercial fruit juices, and fruit spreads. Since fruits, especially berries and grapes, are usually colonized with mold or yeast, they are best avoided too.

6. Avoid nuts, seeds, and beans, at least in the initial phase, as they also harbor a lot of mold.

7. Avoid fermented foods, including those made with soy sauce, miso soup, malt (found in many breakfast cereals), and mushrooms.

8. Avoid tomato sauce, since it is usually full of mold and yeast.

9. Avoid or limit coffee and chocolate, as they are made from beans and often have high mold content. Since tea is made from dried leaves, it may also have a good deal of mold.

10. Avoid bacon, deli meats, sausage, and smoked meats and fish.

Things to Include in a Yeast/Mold-Free Diet:

1. Choose fresh, lean meat and poultry.

2. Choose up to two pieces of fresh fruit a day (avoiding grapes, berries, and melon). Fruits and vegetables should either be peeled or washed carefully.

3. Fresh vegetables of all types.

4. Dairy: Choose organic, low-fat dairy products when feasible.

5. Fresh eggs: Opt for the omega-3 enriched eggs when available; some butter may be okay.

6. Whole grains: Choose barley (not malted), buckwheat, corn, millet, oats, and rice.

7. Beans and peas: Cooked beans, chick peas, and tofu (from soybeans) are usually safe.

8. Choose potatoes and sweet potatoes.

9. Rice cakes and crackers, popcorn, matzoh, and tortillas are usually okay.

10. Beverages: Choose pure spring water, or seltzer. A few ounces of freshly squeezed orange juice may be taken each day.

11. Oils: Choose olive or sesame for cooking; for salads and other uses, choose flax, olive, safflower, sunflower, or walnut oils.

12. For salad dressing, use oil and lemon juice.

13. Seasonings: Basil or other fresh herbs, fresh garlic or onion, can be used.

14. Noodles, pasta, and sauce: Noodles and pasta may be tolerated if the sauce is made from fresh peeled tomatoes, olive oil, and herbs only, and if no cheese is added.

15. Nut butters, and even fruits, may be acceptable as snacks but should not be tried during the initial week of the yeast/mold-free diet.

Supplements in a Yeast-Free Diet

The following supplements are recommended for a yeast-free diet, and most are available at your local health-food store.

- Aged Garlic Extract from Kyolic—Helps fight yeast, strengthens immune system.

- Candex from Pure Essence—Fights candida.

- Caprylic acid—Natural anti-fungal. Mycopryl 680 from T.E. Neesby, Caprylic Acid from Solgar.

- Digestive enzymes. Digestive Aid #34 from Carlson, Omegazyme from Garden of Life, Mega-Zyme from Enzymatic Therapy, Digest Gold from Enzymedica, Ultra Infla-Zyme from American Biologics.

- Olive leaf extract—Olive Leaf Extract from Solaray, Wellness Olive Leaf from Source Naturals.

- Probiotics—Beneficial bacteria. Kyo-Dophilus from Wakunaga, Gi48 from Lane Labs, PB 8 from Nutrition Now, Culturelle from Allergy Research Group, Acidophilus Pearls from Enzymatic Therapy, BioBeads Probiotic Acidophilus from Natrol, All-Flora from New Chapter, DDS-Plus Acidophilus from UAS Labs.

- Tanalbit Plant Tannin from Intensive Nutrition—Intestinal antifungal.

- Vitamins and minerals—To restore health.

CONCLUSION

In another moment down went Alice after it, never
once considering how in the world she was to get
out again. . . . The rabbit hole went straight on like
a tunnel for some way, and then dipped suddenly
down, so suddenly that Alice had not a moment
to think about stopping herself before she found
herself falling down a very deep well.

—Lewis Carroll, *Alice's Adventures in Wonderland,*
Millennium Fulcrum Edition 3.0

The deep well that Alice fell down could easily refer to chronic Lyme disease—although the maze through which all those touched by this disease need to navigate does not feel as much like a wonderland as it does a house of mirrors.

That said, Lyme disease truly is one of the most challenging and controversial medical disorders in the United States today, which is why we offer this guide as a health-empowerment tool.

As Dr. Galland has said, "Learn to know your body and understand your symptoms." It is this body wisdom, and what you know about yourself, that will help guide you and your licensed, Lyme-literate physician in selecting, incorporating, and monitoring the success of the supplements and other integrative choices outlined in this book.

As we mentioned in the Introduction, but wish to affirm here, it is our deepest hope that this guide will provide honest benefits in terms of insights, options, help, and hope to all people who have been touched by the Lyme disease epidemic.

SELECTED
REFERENCES

American Lyme Disease Association. "What is Lyme disease?" www.aldf.com/Lyme.asp

Bayer Environmental Science. The Maxforce Tick Management System. www.maxforcetms.com/maxforce_tms.html

Bock, Steven J. "The integrative treatment of Lyme disease." (Originally appeared in *International Journal of Integrative Medicine,* May/June 1999, no longer published). www.rhinebeckhealth.com

Burrascano, Jr., Joseph. *Advanced Topics in Lyme Disease: Diagnostic Hints and Treatment Guidelines for Lyme and Other Tick-Borne Illnesses.* 15th edition. [monograph] September 2005.

Centers for Disease Control (CDC). "Lyme disease: diagnosis." Nov. 14, 2003. www.cdc.gov/ncidod/dvbid/lyme/diagnosis.htm.

Centers for Disease Control (CDC). "Lyme disease: the bacterium." CDC—Division of Vector-Borne Infectious Diseases, Nov. 14, 2003. www.cdc.gov/ncidod/dvbid/lyme/bburgdorferi.htm.

Centers for Disease Control (CDC). "Lyme disease treatment and prognosis." October 10, 2005. www.cdc.gov/ncidod/dvbid/lyme/ld_humandisease_treatment.htm.

Centers for Disease Control (CDC). "Recommendations for test performance and interpretation from the Second National Conference on Serologic Diagnosis of Lyme Disease." *MMWR: Morbidity and Mortality Weekly Report.* 1995; 44:590-591.

Centers for Disease Control (CDC). "Tick tips: protect your family from Lyme disease." www.cdc.gov/ncidod/dvbid/lyme/spotlight.

Centers for Disease Control (CDC). *Travelers' Health Yellow Book.* Health Information for International Travel.

"Protection against mosquitoes and other arthropods."
www2.ncid.cdc.gov/travel/yb/utils/ybGet.asp?section=
recs&obj=bugs.htm.

Centers for Disease Control (CDC). "Summary of notifiable diseases—United States," 2003. *MMWR: Morbidity
and Mortality Weekly Report.* April 22, 2005.

Colorado Environmental Pesticide Education Program.
Pesticide Fact Sheet No. 206. "Using insect repellents
safely." Reviewed May 2004. http://wsprod.colostate.
edu/cwis79/FactSheets/Sheets/206web.pdf.

Cowden, W. Lee. "Non-pharmacological remedies for
chronic Lyme Borreliosis." Presented at the 11th Annual
Meeting of the Society for Orthomolecular Health-Medicine in San Francisco, CA, February 24–27, 2005.

Crook, William G. *The Yeast Connection.* New York, NY:
Knopf Publishing Group, 1986.

Demarque, Denis, et al, eds. *Pharmacology and Homeopathic Materia Medica.* France: Editions Boiron, 1997.

Environmental Protection Agency (EPA). "How to use insect repellents safely." www.epa.gov/pesticides/health/
mosquitoes/insectrp.htm. April 17, 2002.

Fett, Marc. "What is a Herxheimer?" In: *How to Do the
Oral Salt & Vitamin C Protocol for Lyme Infection.* 2004.
Online monograph: www.fettnet.com/lymestrategies.

Fett, Marc. *Lyme Strategies: Practical Research on Lyme
Infection.* Online monograph: www.fettnet.com/lyme
strategies.

Galland, Leo. *The Fat-Resistance Diet.* New York, NY:
Broadway Books, 2005. www.randomhouse.com/broad-
way/about/faq.html.

Hoffman, Ronald L. *Lyme Disease.* New Canaan, CT:
Keats Publishing, 1994.

Hollins, James (Environmental Protection Agency—
EPA). Personal communication with James Gormley.
February 2006.

Klinghardt, Dietrich. "Lyme disease: A Look Beyond
Antibiotics." January 7, 2005. www.neuraltherapy.com/
word/Lyme1204.doc.

Klinghardt, Dietrich. The Use of Pharmax Nutraceuticals
in the Treatment of Chronic Lyme Disease. (undated, e-
mail: HQ@pharmaxllc.com).

Lang, Denise. *Coping with Lyme Disease,* 3rd edition. New York, NY: Henry Holt (Owl), 2004.

Lyme Disease Foundation. "Lyme disease." www.lyme. org/otherdis/ld.html.

Lyme Disease Network. "Online library." http://library. lymenet.org/domino/file.nsf

LymeNet. Medical Scientific Abstracts. The Lyme Disease Network of NJ, Inc. www.lymenet.org.

NIH National Institute of Allergy and Infectious Diseases. "Looking at Lyme disease." NIAID Research: Antibiotic Therapy. (undated).

North Carolina State University. "Insect repellent products" [Insect Note—ENT/rsc-5]. April 2005. www.ces.ncsu. edu/depts/ent/notes/Urban/repel.htm .

Schmid, Ron. "Diet and recovery from chronic disease." (unpublished)

Stafford, Kirby C. "Tick bite prevention and the use of insect repellents." Connecticut Agricultural Experiment Station. June 2005. www.caes.state.ct.us/FactSheet-Files/Entomology/TickBitePrevention05.pdf

Stricker, Raphael B. "*Lyme disease: the hidden epidemic.*" (Powerpoint Presentation) Presented at the 11th Annual Meeting of the Society for Orthomolecular Health-Medicine, San Francisco, CA, February 24–27, 2005.

STOP. About STOP. www.stopticks.org/about/index.asp.

United States Department of Agriculture (USDA). Patents: 4-Poster. June 29, 2004. www.ars.usda.gov/Business/Business.htm?modecode=62-05-00-00.

U.S. National Institute of Environmental Health Sciences. "Infectious disease: the human costs of our environmental errors." December 17, 2003. http://ehp.niehs.nih. gov/members/2004/112-1/focus.html.

University of Arizona College of Agriculture and Life Sciences. "Insect repellents." May 2004. http://ag.arizona. edu/pubs/insects/az1311.

Vanderhoof-Forschner, Karen. *Everything You Need to Know About Lyme Disease,* 2nd edition. Hoboken, NJ: John Wiley, 2003.

Wormser, Gary P, et al. "Practice guidelines for the treatment of Lyme disease," *Clinical Infectious Diseases,* 2000; 31(Suppl 1):S1–S14.

RESOURCES

American Lyme Disease Foundation
PO Box 466
Lyme, CT 06371
Website: www.aldf.com
E-mail: inquire@aldf.com

Clark Casteel, D.O.M., L.Ac.
Eastern Healing Arts
604 Washington Street A-4
Gainesville, GA 30501
Ph: 1-770-297-0711 or
    1-770-536-2453
Fax: 1-770-297-0711
E-mail: EastNHealingArts@aol.com

Dr. Kathleen Hall
PO Box 1150
Clarkesville, GA 30523
Ph: 1-877-258-3795 or
    1-706-947-1815
Website: www.drkathleenhall.com
E-mail: info@drkathleenhall.com

Foundation for Integrated Medicine
Dr. Leo Galland, Director
133 East 73rd Street
New York, NY 10021
Ph: 1-212-772-3077
Fax: 1-212-794-0170
Website: http://mdheal.org

The Lyme Disease Foundation
P.O. Box 332
Tolland, CT 06084
Ph: 1-860-870-0070
Fax: 1-860-870-0080
Website: www.lyme.org
E-mail: info@lyme.org

The Lyme Disease Network of New Jersey, Inc.
Bill Stolow, President
43 Winton Road
East Brunswick, NJ 08816
Ph: 1-732-238-8579
Fax: 1-732-390-9809
Website: www.lymenet.org
E-mail: bstolow@LymeNet.org

Natural Solutions Foundation
Rima E. Laibow, M.D., Medical Director
88 Batten Road
Croton-on-Hudson, NY 10520
Ph: 1-914-271-6792
Fax: 1-914-730-9805
Website: www.healthfreedomusa.org
E-mail: naturalsolution@optonline.net

Turn the Corner Foundation
15 West 63rd Street, 23A
New York, NY 10023
Ph: 1-212-580-6262
Fax: 1-212-874-3600
Website: www.turnthecorner.org
E-mail: info@turnthecorner.org

Magazines

Let's Live Magazine
Consumer magazine with emphasis on the health benefits of vitamins, minerals, and herbs.

Customer service:
1-800-676-4333
P.O. Box 74908
Los Angeles, CA 90004
Subscriptions: 12 issues per year, $19.95 in the U.S.;
$31.95 outside the U.S.

Physical Magazine
Magazine oriented to body builders and other serious athletes.

Customer service:
1-800-676-4333
P.O. Box 74908
Los Angeles, CA 90004
Subscriptions: 12 issues per year, $19.95 in the U.S.;
$31.95 outside the U.S.

The Nutrition Reporter™ newsletter
Monthly newsletter that summarizes recent medical research on vitamins, minerals, and herbs.

Customer service:
P.O. Box 30246
Tucson, AZ 85751-0246
e-mail: jack@thenutritionreporter.com
www.nutritionreporter.com
Subscriptions: $26 per year (12 issues) in the U.S.; $32 U.S.
or $48 CNC for Canada; $38 for other countries

Websites
James J. Gormley, co-author of *User's Guide to Natural Treatments for Lyme Disease.*

www.jamesgormley.com

Caren Feingold Tishfield, co-author of *User's Guide to Natural Treatments for Lyme Disease.*

www.foodtrainers.net

INDEX

9 781681 628653